Finding Hope and Compassion

Inspiration for Doctors, Nurses, and Other Caregivers Coping with Illness, Disability, or Suffering

Edited by

William P. Beetham, Jr., M.D., Retired
Formerly on Staff of Lahey Clinic and
New England Deaconess Hospital, and
Assistant Professor of Medicine, Harvard Medical School

Ellen B. Ceppetelli, R.N., M.S., C.N.L.
Director Nursing Education
Dartmouth-Hitchcock Medical Center

Carolyn B. Charron, B.S., R.N., O.C.N.
Oncology Nurse, Dana-Farber Cancer Institute, Boston, MA
Former Hospice Nurse, V.N.A. Care, Cambridge, MA

Joseph F. O'Donnell, M.D.
Senior Advising Dean, Director of Community Programs and
Professor of Medicine, Dartmouth Medical School
Former Chief of Oncology, White River Junction V.A. Hospital

Foreword by

Martha Stoddard Holmes, Ph.D.
Associate Professor of Literature and Writing Studies
California State University, San Marcos

Illustrated by

Larry Frates and Herb Packard

Finding Hope and Compassion

Published by:

Gere Publishing

113 Leonard Road

Shutesbury, Massachusetts 01072

www.GerePublishing.com

First Edition

First Printing

Library of Congress Control Number: 2009935244

ISBN 9780974399546

Contents

Foreword

Willingly or not, our lives are lived out in bodies that sicken, hurt, change, and die. On any given day we may find ourselves on a journey through the unstable landscape of illness where the ground can shift without warning as we wait for a diagnosis and a small act of kindness can change the whole day's weather. If illness and disability sometimes threaten to erode our humanity, they are also universal experiences that teach us how to be fully human. The people whose voices fill this book share their richly particular experiences with illness and disability in stories that strike a chord in all of us. *Finding Hope and Compassion* reminds us that our hardest adventures as humans are the source of deep and lasting meaning.

This book contains a wide range of stories about people who are sick or suffering. Diagnosis, treatment, remission, recovery, relapse, and illness management are different for each of us. *Finding Hope and Compassion* acknowledges our human differences while affirming illness and disability as universal life experiences.

This collection offers perspectives on illness from early adulthood through middle age and beyond. The narratives explore not only acute illness, but also chronic illness and disability. Chronic illness is a life reality for more and more of us as improved healthcare lets us live longer than previous generations; as these stories affirm, we can be chronically ill yet living well. Similarly, this collection invites us to consider disabilities not as life disruptions but as integral parts of the full lives we live as vital family and community members, beloved friends, and productive colleagues. If, as Susan Sontag asserts in *Illness as Metaphor*, each of us has a passport in "the kingdom of the ill" as well as "the kingdom of the well," some of us have dual citizenship. We are disabled but healthy; or we shuttle between illness and wellness as we learn to manage bad days and fully enjoy good ones.

The sheer diversity of the stories collected here is crucial to readers who have not yet experienced disability or serious illness and either seek a more intelligent empathy with their loved ones or patients or want to look beyond the present moment to these most universal of human experiences. For readers who find themselves in the midst of illness or newly disabled, the stories offer many opportunities for connection to someone further along the path. The range of genres and lengths included (not just stories, but reflections, poems, and epigraphs) make it an accessible and refreshing book for the hospitalized patient, the doctor on overnight rounds, and the medical student who needs a break from the textbook. For all of us, the collection responds to a need for more varied stories about the life of the body and the human spirit it carries.

Illness and disabilities happen to persons, not just bodies. Each writer in this collection brings a rich stock of other life experiences to their stories. They are husbands and wives; parents, children, and grandchildren; siblings, teachers and students; friends; colleagues in a wide range of work experiences. Perhaps most significantly, they are doctors. We don't expect to hear doctors and medical students offer first-person accounts of illness and disability. The myth of the white coat assumes that doctors are not patients. We may joke about wanting a physician who knows the gap between "a little discomfort" and pain, or knows firsthand what chemotherapy feels like, but the predominant view is that getting sick or developing a disability sidelines a doctor or medical student. The idea that illness experiences confer specialized knowledge, understanding, and compassion that professionals can bring to the practice of medicine still meets with resistance. Drs. Iezzoni, Jamison, Khan, Nutt, and Remen invite us to re-imagine the white coat and its meaning in more imaginative and human ways. Their stories should be required reading for patients, present and future doctors, and medical educators.

Further, while published accounts of illness and disability often include the perspectives of spouses or other family members, sometimes in the form of stories written collaboratively, this book includes a genre we don't often get: the story of an illness told by the patient and by his or her doctor. This fascinating dual perspective may well be the next wave in illness narratives, following Dr. Rita Charon's ethical decision to share with her patients her written accounts of their experiences and enlist their help in "getting it right." The paired narratives in *Finding Hope and Compassion* remind us that illness and disability are relational experiences, deriving their worst and best meanings by the way they shape our interactions with other people. In addition, they give us a wonderful window on the ways that doctors and patients can work together, each contributing specialized and very different knowledge, to create the meaning and relevance of an Illness.

My appreciation for this book and books like it is anything but casual. Years after my first meeting with Drs. Beetham and O'Donnell and shortly after beginning to write this foreword, I was diagnosed with ovarian cancer. As I anxiously surfed the Internet looking not just for information (what did we know? what should I expect? how bad could it be?) but also stories (what happened to you? how is it like and not like what is happening to me?), I inevitably thought about this book and returned to reread its narratives about cancer. Especially when I was trying to be "patient"—waiting for the first oncologist appointment, the surgery, the full diagnosis, and the first session of chemotherapy—I was hungry for stories. I needed help to imagine the best or the worst that could happen and simply to make my illness a territory with familiar outlines and recognizable landmarks, already visualized and thus not quite so scary. Even before that first doctor visit, other people's stories gave me a nodding acquaintance with the language of this new world. I was able to do more than sit, overwhelmed and silent, or thank the doctor for bad news, "habit being so strong," like the narrator of Robert Carver's poem "What the Doctor Said." Above all, other people's stories reminded me that I was not alone. They offered the company and support of fellow travelers in the kingdom of the ill.

Stories are our lifelines in the first few chill days of trying to recognize the lives and bodies we thought we knew as our own. They support us as we learn how to claim illness and disability as parts of lives that are not yet over, in which we are really alive until we take our last breaths. Stories help us make sense of the ending of lives when cure is no longer possible. The stories, poems, and reflections in this book are excellent company for all of these human journeys.

Martha Stoddard Holmes, Ph.D.
Assistant Professor of Literature and Writing Studies
College of Arts and Sciences
California State University San Marcos

Acknowledgments

This publication was made possible by a generous grant from Purdue Pharma L.P.

Thank you to Larry Frates and Herb Packard for their original artwork designed for the book.

A special thank you to Claudia Gere, our literary agent and publisher, for her undying belief, optimism, and perseverance in getting the book published.

Introduction

We cannot always remain young and healthy. Unexpected disability can happen to any of us, anywhere, anytime, changing our lives and the lives of loved ones who share their lives with us. The sick and disabled not only open our eyes to the needs of others, but also remind us what our own lives might be like if we had their condition.

This book is divided into three sections. Section I is entitled, "Love and Compassion." It contains inspirational writing and poetry. Section II, "Inspirational Rea-Life Stories," has true stories about people who are handicapped or have serious illnesses. The stories in this section describe a wide variety of illnesses including 29 different conditions. Each story uses the storyteller's own words as much as possible and includes a brief commentary or introduction by someone knowledgeable about that person's condition. This allows us to see an illness from the viewpoint of those who are sick or disabled or those who care for them. These stories show that we need courage to survive difficult times, that hope and faith count, that living generously means taking risks and reaching out to help others. Each story is complete in itself and can be read individually or one after the other. Section III, "Living Fully," contains inspirational essays and poems and is divided into three smaller sections entitled, "Courage," "Suffering, Compassion, and Nursing," and "Hope and Faith."

Most but not all of the stories in this book have been published before and reveal empathy and compassion. Whenever possible, the stories in Section II include photographs of the people involved, helping us identify with them. When no photographs were available, the stories were illustrated by Herb Packard. Sections I and III are illustrated by Larry Frates with original drawings that have amber overlay.

We all have memories about the good times and bad times in our own lives. It is easy to become so preoccupied with our own lives that we fail to see the needs of others. These stories help us realize that life is a precious gift. It should be enjoyed before it is too late. When faced with severe illness, we suddenly notice the beauty and hidden love all around us that we really have not seen before, as described by Gale Warner and Cheryl Proal.

We become more tolerant, more compassionate, and more aware of the needs of people that we meet in our daily life. Pain and suffering have the power to transform our lives, bringing inner strength and self-renewal.

It takes courage for those struck by unexpected disability to get up and keep going after being knocked down. We can show respect for those who are dependent on others or give comfort to those in pain by simple acts of kindness. Dr. Rachel Remen reminds us that listening, a smile, or a kind word can give someone who is lonely or disabled new hope.

Dr. Howard Spiro of Yale Medical School wrote an enlightening article entitled, "What Is Empathy and Can It Be Taught?" (*Annals of Internal Medicine*, 1992). Empathy is an intimate understanding of someone else's thoughts and feelings. It can renew hope. "You become a friend and not a stranger." Empathy can be strengthened by listening to stories and reading literature, by helping others, and by an awareness of suffering.

When people are sick or dying, they often need spiritual support. In his book, *Anatomy of Hope: How People Prevail in the Face of Illness* Dr. Jerome Groopman shares his thoughts about the importance of hope in sustaining the life of people with chronic or terminal disease. His experience as a cancer specialist and his own episode of disabling back pain taught him how grateful people can be when hope is restored to them. Since there is no easy way for everyone to find hope, physicians and nurses can listen to the emotional and spiritual needs of sick people under their care, seeking additional support from clergy, counselors, and family if necessary.

Faith can give those who reach out for spiritual strength both inner peace and hope, although it does not always supply us with all the answers. Fra Giovanni wrote, "The gloom of the world is but a shadow, behind it, yet within our reach is joy . . . the day breaks and the shadows flee away. Nurture strength of spirit to shield you in sudden misfortune." People are able to endure unbelievable circumstances if only they do not suffer in isolation. It is always comforting to know that we are not alone and are surrounded by love, family and friends.

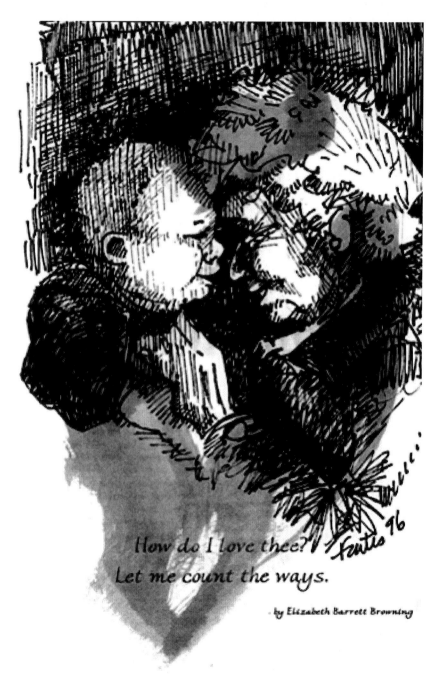

How do I love thee?
Let me count the ways.

by Elizabeth Barrett Browning

Illustrated by Larry Frates

Section I.

Love & Compassion

Share Your Love

By Leo Buscaglia

This beloved American author, teacher, and lecturer shares his joy and enthusiasm for life with us. He believes there are numerous opportunities every day to make someone happy by being kind and by taking the time to listen to other people's needs. His compassion and insights show us how we can love and be loved.

Dr. Buscaglia worked a great deal with handicapped individuals and patients with terminal cancer. He always said his greatest honor was receiving the "Lifetime Achievement Award" from Hospice.

The majority of us lead quiet, unheralded lives as we pass through this world. There will most likely be no ticker-tape parades for us, no monuments created in our honor. But that does not lessen our possible impact, for there are scores of people waiting for someone just like us to come along; people who will appreciate our compassion, our encouragement, who will need our unique talents, who will live a happier life merely because we took the time to share what we had to give.

Too often we underestimate the power of a touch, a smile, a kind word, a listening ear, an honest compliment, or the smallest act of caring; all of which have the potential to turn a life around. It's overwhelming to consider the continuous opportunities there are to make our love felt.

Desiderata

By Max Ehrmann

When Adlai Stevenson, the influential presidential nominee, governor, and U.S. Ambassador to the United Nations, died of a heart attack, he had the following eloquent statement by Max Ehrmann in his coat pocket. It is a list of the essential qualities needed to live a worthwhile life. Desiderata *is the plural form of the Latin word* desideratum *which means something needed and desired.*

Go placidly amid the noise and the haste, and remember what peace there may be in silence. As far as possible, without surrender, be on good terms with all persons. Speak your truth quietly and clearly; and listen to others, even to the dull and the ignorant; they too have their story. Avoid loud and aggressive persons; they are vexatious to the spirit. If you compare yourself with others, you may become vain or bitter, for always there will be greater and lesser persons than yourself.

Enjoy your achievements as well as your plans. Keep interested in your own career, however humble; it is a real possession in the changing fortunes of time. Exercise caution in your business affairs, for the world is full of trickery. But let this not blind you to what virtue there is; many persons strive for high ideals, and everywhere life is full of heroism.

Be yourself. Especially do not feign affection. Neither be cynical about love; for in the face of all aridity and disenchantment, it is as perennial as the grass. Take kindly the counsel of the years, gracefully surrendering the things of youth. Nurture strength of spirit to shield you in sudden misfortune. But do not distress yourself with dark imaginings. Many fears are born of fatigue and loneliness.

Beyond a wholesome discipline, be gentle with yourself. You are a child of the universe no less than the trees and the stars; you have a right to be here. And whether or not it is clear to you, no doubt the universe is unfolding as it should. Therefore be at peace with God, whatever you conceive Him to be. And whatever your labors and aspirations, in the noisy confusion of life, keep peace in your soul. With all its sham, drudgery and broken dreams, it is still a beautiful world. Be cheerful. Strive to be happy.

See Me

By an Unknown Elderly Woman

This vivid poem restores dignity to the life of a neglected elderly woman who needs compassion and respect. It was found after her death among her possessions in the geriatric ward of Ashludie Hospital, near Dundie, Scotland. No information is available concerning who she was or when she died. This poem was read at Clackamus College, Senior Citizen's Day, May 24, 1977.

What do you see, nurses, what do you see?
    Are you thinking, when you look at me—

A crabby old woman, not very wise,
    Uncertain of habit, with far-away eyes.

Who dribbles her food and makes no reply
    When you say in a loud voice, "I do wish you'd try!"

Who seems not to notice the things that you do,
    And forever is losing a stocking or shoe.

Who unresisting or not, lets you do as you will
    With bathing and feeding, the long day to fill.

Is that what you're thinking? Is that what you see?
    Then open your eyes, nurse, you're looking at ME.

I'll tell you who I am, as I sit here so still,
    As I rise at your bidding, as I eat at your will.

I'm a small child of ten with a father and mother,
    Brothers and sisters who love one another;

At twenty-five now I have young of my own
    Who need me to build a secure happy home;

A woman of thirty, my young now grow fast,
    Bound to each other with ties that should last;

At forty my young sons are grown and are gone,
 But my man's beside me to see I don't mourn;

At fifty once more babies play 'round my knee,
 Again we know children, my loved one and me.

Dark days are upon me; my husband is dead.
 I look at the future. I shudder with dread.

For my young are all rearing young of their own,
 And I think of the years and the love that I've known.

I'm an old woman now and nature is cruel;
 'Tis her jest to make old age look like a fool.

The body is crumbled, grace and vigor depart;
 There is now a stone where once I had a heart.

But inside this old carcass a young girl still dwells,
 And now, again, my battered heart swells.

I remember the joys, I remember the pain.
 And I'm loving and living life over again.

I think of the years, all too few, gone too fast,
 And I accept the stark fact that nothing can last.

So open your eyes, nurses, open and see,
 Not a crabby old woman, look closer, nurses—see ME!

What Is Life?

Anonymous

We have been unable to find the author of this quotation, which has been used to inspire patients with terminal cancer in Hospice programs. The joyful message of this quotation helps us realize that life is a precious gift full of opportunity and challenge.

Life is a gift; accept it.

Life is an adventure; dare it.

Life is a duty; complete it.

Life is a promise; fulfill it.

Life is a journey; complete it.

Life is an opportunity; take it.

Life is beauty; praise it.

Life is a challenge; meet it.

Life is a sorrow; overcome it.

Life is costly, care for it.

Life is a tragedy; transcend it.

Life is a mystery; unfold it.

Life is a song, sing it.

Finding Hope & Compassion

If I Had My Life to Live Over

By Nadine Stair

This delightful elderly woman believes that life is a journey. It is full of excitement and there is much to see on the way. Enjoy the trip, for life should be lived as you go along. Take risks! Some opportunities may never come again.

I'd dare to make more mistakes next time.
I'd relax. I would limber up.
I'd be sillier than I have been this trip.
I would take fewer things seriously.
I would take more chances.
I would take more trips.
I would climb more mountains and swim more rivers.
I would eat more ice cream and less beans.
I would perhaps have more actual troubles but I'd have fewer
    imaginary ones.
You see, I'm one of those people who live sensibly and sanely hour
    after hour, day after day.
Oh, I've had my moments, and if I had it to do over again,
    I'd have more of them. In fact, I'd try to have nothing else.
    Just moments.
One after another, instead of living so many years
    ahead of each day.
I've been one of those people who never go anywhere without a
    thermometer, a hot water bottle, a raincoat, and a parachute.
If I had it to do again, I would travel lighter next time.
If I had my life to live over, I would start barefoot earlier in the
    spring and stay that way later in the fall.
I would go to more dances.
I would ride more merry-go-rounds.
I would pick more daisies.

Gale Warner

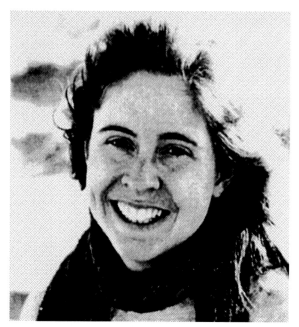

Photo by David Kreger, M.D.

Gale Warner died of non-Hodgkin's lymphoma at the age of 31.

"When people hear they have cancer, they suddenly notice the sweetness of the air, the beauty of trees, the tenderness of loved ones, and are seized by wonder. 'How is it I have been living and not truly seeing this before?' But I have no sense of having let life slip by, no regret for the dreams I did not follow."

– Gale Warner

Section II.

Inspirational Life Stories

Dancing at the Edge of Life

By Gale Warner

Gale Warner was an accomplished poet and journalist who died of lymphoma at age 31. She describes her courageous struggle against cancer in a beautifully written book, Dancing at the Edge of Life, *edited by Dr. David Kreger, her husband.*

The lymphoma caused episodes of fever, chest pain, difficulty breathing, and fatigue. It spread to her liver, lymph nodes in her chest, and other nodes in her body. Gale received intensive chemotherapy and radiation that produced hair loss, nausea, mouth sores, and skin lesions. She developed loss of appetite, constipation, abdominal cramps, sleep disturbance, and mood swings. Low blood cell counts required transfusions. A bone marrow transplant failed.

Gale found spiritual strength in writing and dancing. She urges us to laugh, love, and look for hidden beauty all around us while we have the chance. The following excerpts from Gale's diary describe her feelings at different stages in her illness:

November 29. 1990

When people hear they have cancer, they suddenly notice the sweetness of the air, the, beauty of the trees, the tenderness of loved ones, and are seized by wonder. "How is it I have been living and not truly seeing this before?" But I have no sense of having let life slip by, no regret for the dreams I did not follow. I will keep loving as before, writing as before.

June 3. 1991

This evening, David and I sat on the quarry cliff, the place where we had decided to marry, and looked over the marsh. My breath was squeezed and raspy. I could not tell him I was safe. And yet such a calm came into my spirit as I looked at his beloved face, I said, "If this were the only evening we had left, this would be enough."

June 27. 1991

I'm not confident in the radiation, in my body, in the transplant. This tumor has succeeded in terrifying me with its persistence. What is next?

I am writing for my life, and oh, it is not as easy as it sounds. You can't just snap your fingers and blithely announce, "I want to live," and have a sudden flood of deep inner resources automatically surge through your being. I have to work. I have to unlock the deep desires, the desire of the heart to keep beating, of my brain to keep on flashing and creating, of rivers of blood and lymph to keep on flowing. The demons, the grinning ugly gremlins of despair scuttle out of reach when I whirl around to face them—yet they hold some of the keys.

"So, you're here, you miserable monsters. We have much to discuss! You shrink away on this bright morning, but I know you'll be back!" I have grabbed one key already. One tiny, golden key that unlocks desire and opens me to my natural fullness. Despair says, "You can't change anything!" But I banish it and say, "I am a daughter of the four winds, a child of the moon and rain and sun. I am sister to the whale, the osprey, and the juniper. I belong here. The desires of my kin are my desires. I am a seed that desires to root, to grow, and to blossom."

July 11, 1991

God cannot heal us alone; he needs us as full and willing partners, pulling our own weight. As long as I know I am doing this, genuinely, I can relax and say, "The rest is up to you." This is really what I mean when I say, "My life is in your hands." I mean that I am doing what I can, but know I cannot do anything without the support of all that is sacred and loving. Alone and disconnected, I am small and weak. Loved and noticed, I am large and strong and capable of miraculous things. The guardian angels are there, but they can't help if we ignore them . . . So prayer—humble, undemanding, simple prayer—is always worth it.

November 28. 1991

Sorrow is as natural and beautiful as joy: it is only right to grieve at the death of a river, or a child, or a worthy idea. It is right—even somehow magnificent—to weep for your own death. In fact, it feels like an achievement. A year ago, I would not have known how to express this sadness. Now I am both drained, and left with a sense of curious peace.

December 17. 1991

Dear loved ones,

This is a difficult letter to write. Five days ago we learned that my body is again experiencing a major setback. I have several new tumors growing in my liver and a number of large nodes scattered throughout my body. One of the liver tumors is large enough to be causing a number of symptoms, including nightly fevers and pain in my ribs and pelvis. The pain in the pelvis that bothers me most makes it difficult for me to walk (although I still can). I am taking pain medications now, however, and am glad to say that I am doing better than a few days ago.

In short, the transplant did not work. We always knew this was a possibility, but we had hoped for the best, and discovering these new tumors only six days after leaving the hospital was a blow, to say the least. My situation is now quite different and we are adjusting ourselves to a new reality very quickly. I must hurry to tell you that I am basically fine, and that on the deepest levels my soul is not panicked. David and I have been engaged in a wonderful, difficult, joyous process of talking, crying, philosophizing, laughing, and grieving. My faith and my belief systems are rock-solid, my life feels well-ordered, with very little unfinished business, and my spiritual bags are packed. Even if I must leave soon, I think I will be able to make myself ready to go. Of course I would still prefer to stay, and as long as life remains pleasant and interesting to me, as it definitely still is, I will do all I can to hang on.

I already feel your complete support and love, and I will love to hear your thoughts and feelings, your reflections, when you are ready to speak them.

Much love, Gale

Gale died on December 26, 1991, three hours after she whispered the words to "Lord of the Dance," "Wondrous Love," and then "Amazing Grace" beneath her oxygen mask, surrounded by family and friends who sang with her. After a long struggle, her rapid breathing had quieted down and she died peacefully in bed.

My Journey Back to Life

By Lance Armstrong

Cancer survivor Lance Armstrong won the grueling 21-day, 2,288-mile Tour de France bike race seven times in a row starting in 1999. This race is one of the world's most strenuous athletic events. He also triumphed over testicular cancer that was diagnosed three years before his first Tour de France victory. The cancer had spread to his abdomen, lungs, and brain, and he was given a 40 percent chance of survival. The birth of his son, Luke, conceived with sperm that Armstrong banked before starting cancer treatment, is another joyful miracle for Lance and his wife Kristin. The Lance Armstrong Foundation was established in 1997 to raise funds for cancer awareness and research. The following inspiring excerpts are taken from his book, It's Not About the Bike: My Journey Back to Life. *Armstrong's book was written with Sally Jenkins.*

There are angels on this earth and they come in subtle forms, and I decided that LaTrice Haney was one of them. Outwardly, she looked like just another efficient, clipboard-and-syringe-wielding nurse in a starched outfit. She worked extremely long days and nights, and on her off hours she went home to her husband, Randy, a truck driver, and their two children, Taylor, aged seven, and Morgan, four. But if she was tired, she never seemed it. She struck me as a woman utterly lacking in ordinary resentments, sure of her responsibilities and blessings and unwavering in her administering of care, and if that wasn't angelic behavior, I don't know what was.

Often I'd be alone in the late afternoons and evenings except for LaTrice, and if I had the strength, we'd talk seriously. With most people I was shy and terse, but I found myself talking to LaTrice, maybe because she was so gentle-spoken and expressive herself. LaTrice was only in her late 20s, a pretty young woman with a coffee-and-cream complexion, but she had self-possession and perception beyond her years. While other people our age were out nightclubbing, she was already the head nurse for the oncology research unit. I wondered why she did it. "My satisfaction is to make it a little easier for people," she said.

She asked me about cycling, and I found myself telling her about the bike with a sense of pleasure I hadn't realized I possessed. "How did you start riding?" she asked me. I told her about my first bikes, and the early sense of liberation, and that cycling was all I had done since I was 16. I talked about my various teammates over the years, about their humor and selflessness, and I talked about my mother, and what she had meant to me.

I told her what cycling had given me, the tours of Europe and the extraordinary education, and the wealth. I showed her a picture of my house, with pride, and invited her to come visit, and I showed· her snapshots of my cycling career. She leafed through the images of my racing across the backdrops of France, Italy, and Spain, and she'd point to a picture and ask, "Where are you here?"

I confided that I was worried about my sponsor, Cofidis, and explained the difficulty I was having with them. I told her I felt pressured. "I need to stay in shape, I need to stay in shape," I said over and over again.

"Lance, listen to your body," she said gently. "I know your mind wants to run away. I know it's saying to you, 'Hey, let's go ride.' But listen to your body. Let it rest."

I described my bike, the elegant high performance of the ultralight tubing and aerodynamic wheels. I told her how much each piece cost, and weighed, and what its purpose was. I explained how a bike could be broken down so I could practically carry it in my pocket, and that I knew every part and bit of it so intimately that I could adjust it in a matter of moments.

I explained that a bike has to fit your body, and that at times I felt melded to it. The lighter the frame, the more responsive it is, and my racing bike weighed just 18 pounds. Wheels exert centrifugal force on the bike itself, I told her. The more centrifugal force, the more momentum. It was the essential building block of speed. "There are 32 spokes in a wheel," I said. Quick-release levers allow you to pop the wheel out and change it quickly, and my crew could fix a flat tire in less than 10 seconds.

"Don't you get tired of leaning over like that?" she asked.

Yes, I said, until my back ached like it was broken, but that was the price of speed. The handlebars are only as wide as the rider's shoulders, I explained, and they curve downward in half-moons so you can assume an aerodynamic stance on the bike.

"Why do you ride on those little seats?" she asked.

The seat is narrow, contoured to the anatomy, and the reason is that when you are on it for six hours at a time, you don't want anything to chafe your legs. Better a hard seat than the torture of saddle sores. Even the clothes have a purpose. They are flimsy for a reason: to mold to the body because you have to wear them in weather that ranges from hot to hail. Basically, they're a second skin. The shorts have a chamois padded seat, and the stitches are recessed to avoid rash.

When I had nothing left to tell LaTrice about the bike, I told her about the wind. I described how it felt in my face and in my hair. I told her about being in the open air, with the views of soaring Alps, and the glimmer of valley lakes in the distance. Sometimes the wind blew as if it were my personal friend, sometimes as if it were my bitter enemy, sometimes as if it were the hand of God pushing me along. I described the full sail of a mountain descent, gliding on two wheels only an inch wide.

"You're just out there, free," I said.

"You love it," she said.

"Yeah?" I said.

"Oh, I see it in your eyes," she said.

I understood that LaTrice was an angel one evening late in my last cycle of chemo. I lay on my side, dozing on and off, watching the steady, clear drip-drip of the chemo as it slid into my veins. LaTrice sat with me, keeping me company, even though I was barely able to talk.

"What do you think, LaTrice?" I asked, whispering. "Am I going to pull through this?"

"Yeah," she said. "Yeah, you are."

"I hope you're right," I said, and closed my eyes again.

LaTrice leaned over to me.

"Lance," she said softly, "I hope someday to be just a figment of your imagination. I'm not here to be in your life for the rest of your life. After you leave here, I hope I never see you ever again. When you're cured, hey, let me see you in the papers, on TV, but not back here. I hope to help you at the time you need me, and then I hope I'll be gone. You'll say, 'Who was that nurse back in Indiana? Did I dream her?'"

It was one of the single loveliest things anyone has ever said to me. And I will always remember every blessed word.

On December 13, 1996, I took my last chemo treatment. It was almost time to go home.

Shortly before I received the final dose of VIP, Craig Nichols came by to see me. He wanted to talk with me about the larger implications of cancer. He wanted to talk about "the obligation of the cured."

It was a subject I had become deeply immersed in. I had said to Nichols and to LaTrice many times over the last three months, "People need to know about this." As I went through therapy, I felt increasing companionship with my fellow patients. Often I was too sick for much socializing, but one afternoon LaTrice asked me to go to the children's ward to talk to a young boy who was about to start his first cycle. He was scared and self-conscious, just like me. I visited with him for a while, and I told him, "I've been so sick. But I'm getting better." Then I showed him my driver's license.

In the midst of chemo, my license had expired. I could have put off renewing it until I felt better and had grown some hair back, but I decided not to. I pulled on some sweatclothes and hauled myself down to the Department of Motor Vehicles, and stood in front of the camera. I was completely bald, with no eyelashes or eyebrows, and my skin was the color of a pigeon's underbelly. But I looked into the lens, and I smiled.

"I wanted this picture so that when I got better, I would never forget how sick I've been," I said. "You have to fight."

After that, LaTrice asked me to speak with other patients more and more often. It seemed to help them to know that an athlete was fighting the fight alongside them. One afternoon LaTrice pointed out that I was still asking her questions, but the nature of them had changed. At first, the questions I had asked were strictly about myself, my own treatments, my doses, my particular problems. Now I asked about other people. I was startled to read that eight million Americans were living with some form of cancer; how could I possibly feel like mine was an isolated problem? "Can you believe how many people have this?" I asked LaTrice.

"You've changed," she said, approvingly. "You're going global."

Dr. Nichols told me that there was every sign now that I was going to be among the lucky ones who cheated the disease. He said that as my health improved, I might feel that I had a larger purpose than just myself. Cancer could be an opportunity as well as a responsibility. Dr. Nichols had seen all kinds of cancer patients become dedicated activists against the disease, and he hoped I would be one of them.

I hoped so, too. I was beginning to see cancer as something that I was given for the good of others. I wanted to launch a foundation, and I asked Dr. Nichols for some suggestions about what it might accomplish. I wasn't yet clear on what the exact purpose of the organization would be; all I knew was that I felt I had a mission to serve others that I'd never had before, and I took it more seriously than anything in the world.

I had a new sense of purpose, and it had nothing to do with my recognition and exploits on a bike. Some people won't understand this, but I no longer felt that it was my role in life to be a cyclist. Maybe my role was to be a cancer survivor.

Rachel Naomi Remen, M.D.

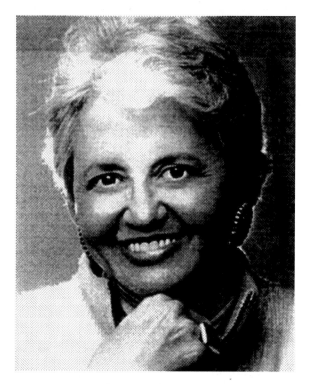

Photograph © Helen Marcus 1996

"Who taught you all this, Doctor?"
The reply came promptly: "Suffering."

– Albert Camus, *The Plague*

Just Listen

By Rachel Naomi Remen, M.D.

Dr. Rachel Remen's book, Kitchen Table Wisdom, *is full of personal stories about wisdom, listening, and compassion. She has Crohn's disease and sees life from the unusual perspective of a well-trained physician, a patient with a long history of chronic disease, and a counselor sensitive to emotional and spiritual needs. Her intestinal disease started at age fifteen and has required multiple operations, including an ileostomy.*

As a child, she was raised in a family with nine physicians and three nurses that represented the objective scientific viewpoint. It was assumed that she would become a doctor when she grew up. Rachel's grandfather also had a major influence on her life. He was an orthodox rabbi and scholar. One of Rachel's fondest childhood memories was spending Sunday afternoons with her beloved grandfather. His blessings and sacred teachings left her with a lasting desire to support the emotional and spiritual needs of other people.

Just listening to other people with genuine concern is comforting. The following quotations by Rachel Remen reveal ways that we can listen to other people:

I suspect that the most basic and powerful way to connect to another person is to listen. Just listen. Perhaps the most important thing we ever give each other is our attention. And especially if it's given from the heart. When people are talking, there's no need to do anything but receive them. Just take them in. Listen to what they are saying. Care about it. Most times caring about it is even more important than understanding it. Most of us don't value ourselves or love enough to know this. It has taken me a long time to believe in the power of simply saying, "I'm so sorry," when someone is in pain. And meaning it.

One of my patients told me that when she tried to tell her story, people often interrupted to tell her that they once had something just like that happen to them. Subtly her pain became a story about themselves. Eventually she stopped talking to most people. It was just too lonely. We connect through listening. When we interrupt what someone is saying to let them know that we understand, we move the focus of attention to ourselves. When we listen, they know we care. Many people with cancer talk about the relief of having someone just listen.

I have even learned to respond to someone crying by just listening. In the old days I used to reach for the tissues, until I realized that passing a person a tissue may be just another way to shut them down, to take them out of their experience of sadness and grief. Now I just listen. When they have cried all they need to cry, they find me there with them.

This simple thing has not been that easy to learn. It certainly went against everything I had been taught since I was very young. I thought people listened only because they were too timid to speak or did not know the answer. A loving silence often has far more power to heal and to connect than the most well-intentioned words.

Bring the Words Forward

By Joshua Lee, M.D.

Dr. Lee is an internist, assistant professor of medicine, and advisor to the Clinical Information Systems Division at Dartmouth Medical School. The following poem appeared in the "Poet on Call" feature in the Fall 2001 issue of Dartmouth Medicine:

Hearing stories is the essence of my work…

I'm afraid I might miss important details.

To share everyday life is so poignant…

Communication is the root of medicine…

We need to make it safe for people to tell their stories

in their own voices, instead of distorting them

into a physician's voice. So much medicine is translation

of the patient's word into the doctor's.

You tend to pigeon-hole a certain word into a complaint

you know a diagnosis for. You have to balance

your knowledge and the patient's individual needs.

You have to go to the patients

and bring their words forward.

Peter Selwyn, M.D.

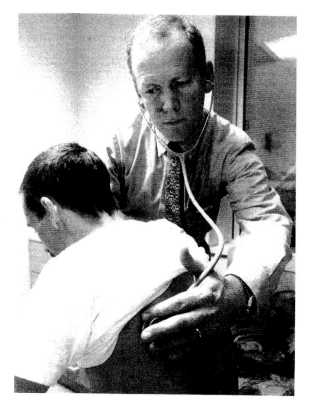

Photo by ENELYSION/George Ruhe

Dr. Peter Selwyn examines a patient at Leeway, a skilled nursing facility in New Haven, Connecticut, for people with AIDS.

Simple Acts of Nurturing

By Peter Selwyn, M.D.

During his internship at the Montefiore Medical Center in the Bronx and subsequent medical appointments, Dr. Selwyn observed the AIDS epidemic among many injection-drug users. He describes these patients and their deaths at an early age in his book Surviving the Fall: The Personal Journey of an AIDS Doctor. *These experiences helped him learn how to grieve for his own father's probable suicide at an early age. Dr. Selwyn served as the associate director of the Yale AIDS Program and then became chairman of the Department of Family Medicine at the Montefiore Medical Center, Albert Einstein College of Medicine. The excerpt that follows is taken from his book and has also been published in the* Winter 1999 issue of the Harvard Medical Alumni Bulletin. *It shows how just listening can give comfort and transform behavior.*

One of my favorite patients was Betty, a 33-year-old Puerto Rican woman whom I first met because she was causing such behavior problems at the methadone clinic that her counselor was ready to terminate her from the program. She was loud, demanding, articulate, and extremely manipulative, and she was an expert at making everyone run around at cross purposes while she sat calmly in the eye of the storm—an "egg beater," as we called such patients. It was apparent from the moment I met her that Betty was also smart, funny, suspicious and, most of all, terrified about her illness and what she feared it would do to her. Betty's 10-year-old daughter, whom she had entrusted to her mother's care, was starting to show some early signs of preadolescent troublemaking in school.

Betty had also had some recent problems with cocaine use. She was afraid that she might be kicked off the methadone program and have to go back to supporting her heroin addiction by working the streets near Hunt's Point Terminal Market in the southeast Bronx. After meeting together with her counselor and the program administrator, we made a deal: we would write up a contract specifying what behavior would and would not be tolerated, as well as the obligation of the program to retain her in treatment as long as she complied with her part of the agreement. It was decided that I would continue to be her doctor—that I would, in fact, be the only medical person she would interact with to avoid further miscommunication.

This agreement worked remarkably well over the next several months. Betty's behavior improved, the frequency of her cocaine-positive urines decreased, and there were fewer complaints about her from clinic staff. One day, however, she became sick. This was in the years before prophylaxis against pneumocystis carinii pneumonia had become standard, and PCP was still the most common illness and cause of death among AIDS patients (now it's almost completely preventable).

Betty had noticed a mild cough for a couple of weeks, along with some slowly progressive shortness of breath. Finally, she was unable even to walk upstairs to get to her apartment or to perform even minimal housework without having to sit down to rest.

She was admitted to the hospital with what looked like a classic case of PCP, and after a few days began to respond to the IV therapy. At that point, however, she became more and more angry and abusive with the nursing staff, accusing them of withholding her methadone or diluting it, and finding fault with even the most trivial details of the hospital routine. The floor nursing staff, who had not known Betty before she had become ill, quickly assessed her as another foul-mouthed drug addict. In the passive-aggressive ways that hospital staff members sometimes react when they don't like a patient, they began to put up their own barriers against her.

Finally, even these defenses were no longer working, and the head nurse asked me to come up to the floor to speak to Betty, "*your* patient," she emphasized, as if to distance herself even further from Betty's distasteful behavior. When I got off the elevator, I was met with a trio of floor nurses, all experienced caregivers, who smiled as they greeted me but could not fully conceal their disgusted conviction that it was somehow my fault that such a patient should exist to make their lives so miserable.

This was a response that I had gotten used to in the hospital. Over the years I had become identified as that doctor in the methadone program who took care of all "those" drug addicts. Being the physician for this large group of drug users meant being tainted by some of the same negative associations that were directed toward the patients themselves.

Although my interactions with nurses and my physician colleagues at the hospital were, in general, excellent, at times I felt that some of them would prefer never to have to deal with me or my difficult and demanding patients again. A friend of mine once told me of a Department of Medicine administrative meeting in the hospital at which someone brought up a problem that had occurred in the ER the night before. A drunken and disheveled homeless patient had shown up and started acting abusively toward the nursing staff. Someone else at the meeting then joked, to everyone's amusement, "Oh, it must have been one of Peter Selwyn's patients."

There was an unspoken double standard in the hospital, which often made it very frustrating trying to schedule certain tests or have procedures performed for patients from the methadone program. On a rare occasion, someone would come right out and declare a hatred for drug addicts or an opinion that they didn't deserve the best care. The chief of one of the non-invasive diagnostic testing services once told me, in perverse ignorance of basic infection control, that he didn't want his equipment contaminated by our patients, and a few surgeons refused outright to operate on our patients with AIDS. More often though, these prejudices were expressed subtly—we were made to feel as though we were begging for crumbs, always having to go to the end of the line.

Of course, it didn't help when our patients refused to cooperate with a procedure or failed to show up for an appointment that we had pleaded for. These transgressions only served to confirm the hospital staff's prejudices and left us feeling foolish, caught in the middle. Sometimes it was even worse, like the time I cajoled the staff at the Family Health Center, my former training site, to let me bring over some of my pregnant patients from the methadone program to have sonograms done there. This was before the Family Health Center itself became a major site for providing HIV care in the local community, and the staff members were still wary because they hadn't yet seen many drug-addicted patients with AIDS. They finally agreed, but one of the first patients I sent over promptly stole a staff member's pocketbook that had been left in a drawer in the examining room.

On the day that the head nurse had asked me to come speak with Betty, I went to the end of the hall to the single isolation room where she was being kept due to her boisterous behavior. When I opened the door, I found that the drawers of her nightstand had been emptied on the floor and her bedclothes flung wildly about the room. Betty stood by the side of her bed, holding her IV pole like Neptune holding his trident, as if she were daring me to come into the room.

I walked in and asked her permission to sit on the edge of the bed. She launched into a five-minute tirade about the injustices she had suffered at the hands of the floor nurse. "I never get my methadone on time, plus they're cutting it with something. Whenever I call they never come, and this food tastes like they're trying to poison me, and no one tells me a god-damned thing about what is going on." My first impulse was to stop her and point out that each accusation she was making was either untrue or explainable by the inscrutable logic of hospital routine. But something made me hold back. I simply sat and listened to what she had to say. After she was finished, she looked at me quizzically, expecting me to respond. I simply looked back at her and nodded, waiting for her to go on.

Betty took a Kleenex box and threw it across the room, explaining that she was tired of being treated like a dirty junkie. I nodded again, and she responded by sliding her breakfast tray over onto the floor with a clash of silverware, her orange juice spilling into a slowly widening circle on the linoleum tiles. I continued to sit, wordless, simply being present.

Finally, when she had run out of things to complain about, I said quietly, "I think I would be pretty upset too if I had just been diagnosed with PCP and was worried about how long I was going to live." Betty looked at me, and then immediately started to cry, continuing for ten minutes, inconsolable, going through half of the Kleenex box, which I had placed back on her bed next to her. When she was finished crying, she looked up at me and began to talk about her real fears of dying, of losing her daughter, of being rejected by her mother's family. We talked for another half-hour while I acknowledged her fears and told her that we would work with her to address them. We also talked about how she would do a lot better and be more likely to get what she wanted if she behaved herself on the unit. On my way out, I told the head nurse that I thought things would start to get better.

Within two days, the same nurses who had been looking for ex-cuses to get Betty to sign herself out of the hospital against medical advice were now going to the coffee shop to get doughnuts for her on their lunch breaks. It was a miraculous transformation, and it taught me, more than any other experience, the importance of simply being there for patients, as a sympathetic companion, not as a judge, commentator, or rescuer. I could have stopped Betty's diatribe and bluntly informed her that her behavior was unacceptable, probably provoking her to act out even more and leave the hospital. Or I could have simply withdrawn myself and told her that I could not help her as long as she acted this way. None of these responses would have resulted in a meaningful solution to the problem of Betty's be-havior, and her unresolved fears and conflicts would have erupted in some other manner, probably in a short period of time. I was reminded of the wisdom of one of my first teachers in medical school, a silver-haired emeritus professor of medicine at Harvard, who gave the sage advice that I have always tried to remember at times like this: "Don't just do something, sit there!"

Betty went on to recover fully from PCP and became very involved in her follow-up medical care. She traveled around the Bronx with a waist pack full of her medication bottles, a schedule for each dose, and a programmable alarm clock that went off to alert her when it was time for her next pill. Before she had been discharged from the hospital, she had told her mother that she had AIDS; her mother embraced her lovingly and pledged to continue to take care of her and her daughter. Betty also regained her wry, mordant sense of humor. When a young emergency room intern asked her during a routine exam whether she had any health problems, she replied, "No, honey. Aside from having AIDS, I am really very healthy."

Betty and I had an easy, joking relationship, and we genuinely liked each other. I remember one time when a stethoscope disappeared in the clinic and the rumor was that a patient had taken it. Betty told me that she didn't know anything about it. I believed her, but she kept insisting, "But Dr. Selwyn, I don't want you to think that I'm a thief!" I laughed and replied, "But Betty, I know you're a thief, and I still love you," and gave her a hug.

Betty's last illness came quickly, and she became rapidly demented and unable to walk over a period of weeks. The rapidity of this course suggested to us that she had one of the more devastating brain infections of AIDS, progressive multi-focal leukoencephalopathy (PML), instead of the more common, indolent dementia associated with AIDS itself. There was no treatment for PML—even now, treatment is marginally effective at best—and, mercifully, patients usually did not survive very long after they had become afflicted. The last time I saw Betty alive, she was propped up in her hospital bed, a teddy bear at her side, her arms and legs twitching in little involuntary jerks. I went into her room, sat by her bed and began, on a sudden impulse, to feed her with a spoon from her tray.

I felt suddenly as if this were the most important thing I could do for her at that moment, though I had a distinctly uncomfortable feeling that it would be embarrassing for me if a group of my colleagues were suddenly to come by and see me feeding her. (How odd that such a simple act of nurturing should seem so out of place for a physician.) I fed Betty some Cream of Wheat, which she slurped up eagerly, reminding me of one of my daughters. I wiped the small dribble of Cream of Wheat from her lower lip with the spoon in the same way that I had done so many times at home. Then I held her hand, sat with her, said goodbye, and left. Once again, I realized with Betty that one of the most important services I could offer as a physician had more to do with being there than anything else.

At her funeral, Betty was laid out in a delicate white lace dress. She looked like an angel as I looked down at her in an open casket. Her daughter sat on a chair in the front row next to her grandmother, her hair tied up in a tight knot in the back, swinging her legs back and forth slowly, her toes almost touching the floor. I looked at her and hoped that she would have the same yearning and zest for life that her mother had. Betty truly helped me to understand what it means to embrace life, and to see that the work we do and the impact we have in the world are measured only, finally, in the people whose lives we touch.

Your Son Is Dying

By Joseph O'Neil, M.D.

AIDS (acquired immunodeficiency syndrome) is a dreaded, epidemic disease that has caused widespread fear and fatality. It is due to HIV infection (the human immunodeficiency virus). People may develop a temporary flu-like syndrome soon after being infected by HIV. Often this is the only symptom an infected person has until years later. The first signs of AIDS appear when the immune system fails and helper T-cells, which defend against infection, are depleted. Eventually tumors and opportunistic infections that usually do not cause disease in normal people become serious threats to survival.

The lives of those affected by AIDS have been dramatically changed in ways that are difficult to imagine. They have endured pain and suffering due to weight loss, fever, fatigue, swollen lymph nodes, purple Kaposi sarcoma skin tumors, neurologic disorders, pneumonia, gastrointestinal disease, and depression.

Dying people may be able to tolerate incredible suffering when surrounded by family and friends after realizing that they are loved and not alone. However, it is very difficult for some family members to recognize and then accept the reality of impending death in a loved one as described by Joseph O'Neil. O'Neil was a medical student caring for a young AIDS patient at the San Francisco General Hospital when he decided the patient and family should be drawn closer together now that the moment of death was near for his patient.

This oral history is based on an interview and shows how a medical student dealt with tragedy by taking a worthwhile risk.

He was very sick; he was wasted. He was paraplegic and in just awful pain. He was a gay man living in San Francisco; his parents lived in Florida. They came out in total denial of what was going on. They loved this guy, their son, passionately . . . and all they wanted to do was fix everything. And they wanted the best doctors, the best that money could buy. "And what does Dr. Volberding say about this?" and "What does Dr. So-and-So . . . ?" I mean every kind of controlling behavior. "He wanted chocolate pudding, and they sent peach pudding. I'm going to call the head of the hospital." They were very hard to deal with. And here I am, this medical student, working with a resident who wasn't even paying that much attention to him because he was no longer an interesting case. And the patient was very much the same way . . . "The room's too bright," "I asked for water, and I didn't get ice in it, and I wanted ice . . . " And meanwhile here's like this skinny, dying young man who's worrying about the flavor of his pudding—you know, I mean the whole thing was wrong.

I remember this; this is where I really learned something about doctoring from him. One morning I was just talking with him and sort of listening to him, and he looked me in the eye and said, "Am I going to die?" And I said, "Yes, you are going to die." And he said "When?" and I said, "Very soon." And he said, "Oh, do my parents know?" And I said, "I think they do, but have you talked with them about it?" And he said, "No, I couldn't talk with them about it. It's too hard. I couldn't talk about it." And I said, "When your parents get here today, you have the nurse page me, and I'll come." And about an hour later we were rounding, and I got paged by the nurse saying they were there.

I came back down and walked in the room, and they were just doing all this stuff. And the whole time—this had been going on for three weeks—I had never seen one of his parents touch him, lay hands on him. I mean, they did everything but. They were running around fixing the blinds, I remember they were fixing the blinds in the room. And I went out and brought in chairs, these folding chairs, and I set up chairs around his bed, and I said, "Stop it." And I mean, there was just me, no nurse, no one else, just me, this little medical student, you know. And I said, "Sit down. We have something very important to discuss here." And so they sat down, and I said, "What we have to discuss is the fact that your son is dying." And I said, "I just want to talk about it. So I'll leave the room if you want, but this is what is happening. There's nothing more we're going to do. Your son is dying, and you really need to spend some time with him."

And I remember his parents, they started crying. And they got up, and they held him, and in three weeks they had never touched him. And I left them, and I said, "You have to say good-bye. It doesn't matter what he's eating. It matters that you spend some time together." I was on call that night. Maybe two hours after they left, he died.

Cheryl Proal

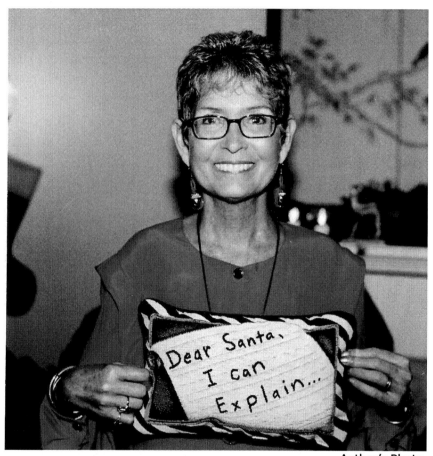

Author's Photo

Cheryl's message is simple. "I know I have my limitations, but I love the fact that I still try. And there are wonderful days like today, with the bright-colored leaves swirling around my feet and the sky the most breathtaking color blue. On a glorious day like this, how could anything possibly be wrong?"

Pain Is Inevitable, Misery Is Optional

By Cheryl Proal
Introduction by William Beetham, Jr., M.D.

I will always remember Cheryl Proal who was under my care for about 15 years prior to my retirement. She has systemic Lupus, which is an immune disorder, and osteonecrosis that required extensive surgery and replacement of multiple joints. Her enthusiasm and cheerfulness, in spite of her limitations, made everyone who knew her feel better. She made the most of her life by setting new goals within her reach.

The October 1996 issue of Guideposts *contains a quotation by an unknown author in a story by Arthur Gordon; "Pain is inevitable; misery is optional." Pain is a reality of life, but misery is an attitude that can be changed by a conscious effort. Cheryl refused to accept misery and tried to live her life fully, supported by family, friends, and spiritual strength.*

I was diagnosed with lupus when I was 19 years old, a sophomore in college, and illness, medications, doctors, and hospitals have been an unwelcome yet integral part of my life for almost 30 years. In many ways, it's difficult to remember what I was like before the onset of my illness, before it interrupted and often ended my dreams and expectations I envisioned for my future. And yet, despite many disappointments and struggles, I can honestly say my life has been truly happy, with blessings too many to count.

For many years I kept a quote from astrophysicist Stephen W. Hawking, who is severely crippled with ALS, also known as Lou Gehrig's disease. Reading it and touching it so often, it's long since "tattered away." To me, his philosophy says it all and so, to paraphrase him: it is not as though I was given two choices in life, one an easy, uncomplicated path and the other a much more difficult road to travel and thereby opted for the latter. I simply dealt with what was offered me and went on.

I'm not fully aware of how or why I maintain my positive, upbeat attitude except to say that, with the exception of my illness, life has treated me with kindness. I've had a loving, supportive, and nurturing family and friendships that both sustain and enrich my life. I've never faced my difficulties alone, but always with people who love me by my side. Furthermore, although I would give almost anything not to have had lupus as my daily companion, I also know with total certainty that facing illness has made me a "nicer" person . . . more compassionate, less judgmental, more empathetic and tolerant of others' weaknesses and shortcomings.

Living with chronic pain continues to be a difficult task to master and I'm sure a "good" day for me would be a "bad" day for someone else. In dealing with pain and subsequent limitations, I try to find balance in my day-to-day life, pushing myself to get up and get moving, just do something, function, participate, when it would be so much easier not to. However, I also allow myself the choice of staying in bed when I need to and I no longer make excuses for going to bed at 8:00 p.m. There are, of course, those times, though rare (thankfully), when the blues hit. I do not wallow in melancholia, but sometimes a good cleansing cry will help and holding my pets in my arms guarantees I'll be smiling soon.

Throughout my illness I have encountered symptoms numerable and varied, joint and muscle pain, nephritis, transient ischemic attacks, muscle atrophy to the point that I could no longer feed or dress myself. At age 28, I lost the job I loved as a flight attendant, I weighed 86 lbs at 5'8", had lost most of my hair, and relied on my parents for even the most simple of tasks—bathing me and cutting my food. I had a bout with pericarditis as well as an emergency surgery on my throat resulting in a vocal cord injury that has left me with a raspy yet memorable voice. Most people meeting me for the first time assume I have a terrible cold and on the phone they call me "sir."

In 1979, I moved to Massachusetts and had the immeasurable good fortune to meet Dr. William Beetham, my rheumatologist. Together, in 1980, we finally weaned me from steroids and controlled flare-ups with a variety of non-steroidal anti-inflammatory meds—Motrin, Naprosyn, Plaquenil and an immune suppressive medication (Imuran). Over many years of treatment by Dr. B, he monitored me closely and oversaw all aspects of my condition, directing me to whatever specialist I needed at the time. I jokingly told him, "I never have to worry about my health because you worry for me."

As my lupus and general health improved, Dr. B and I faced a new set of problems . . . osteonecrosis, precipitated by lupus and long-time steroid use, necessitated replacement of many joints. In 1982, at age 33, I had both my hips replaced; in 1984 my left shoulder replaced; 1986 right shoulder replacement; 1992 replacement of my right hip again with bone grafting; and in 1993 I had both my knees replaced at the same time.

How am I doing? I must admit I thoroughly enjoy setting off the metal detectors at airports! On a more serious note, these surgeries have certainly been a blessing, enabling me to be self-sufficient and providing a degree of mobility that would not have been possible otherwise. Without question, the surgeries have made me better, but they can never make me what I used to be. I accept that and am grateful for what I do have rather than being maudlin over what I've lost.

I can't swim anymore. I swam in competition as a young woman, but my arms no longer go around 360 degrees. And yet, I'm always first in the water and the "doggie paddle" works just fine.

What can I do? I work part-time in a job I love; I own my own home, and delight in cooking and entertaining. I don't ride a bike or play racquetball, but I can lose myself for hours when I'm working on crafts. A few years ago, on a trip to the Caribbean, I rode a horse for the first time in years. Getting me on and off was a struggle, but I did it. When I told Dr. B the story, he stopped short, praised me for my enthusiasm, and told me never to do that again!

I guess that's what it's all about. I know I have my limitations, but I love the fact that I still try. And there are wonderful days like today, with the brightly colored leaves swirling around my feet and the sky the most breathtaking color blue. On a glorious day like this, how could anything possibly be wrong?

On Being a Patient—The Patient-Doctor

By Muhammad Asim Khan, M.D.

Dr. Muhammad Asim Khan is a rheumatologist at Case Western Reserve University School of Medicine, who shares with us his personal experience with ankylosing spondylitis, heart disease, and cancer of the kidney.

Ankylosing spondylitis can be a very disabling disease causing inflammation in many different parts of the body such as the joints, heart, and spine. It is a chronic systemic inflammatory disease characterized by arthritic changes in the sacroiliac joints and, to a varying degree, arthritis of the spine, causing limitation of motion in the back. In late stages it may cause flexion deformities of the spine, hips, and knees. Ankylosing spondylitis may also cause fatigue, morning stiffness, iritis, heart involvement (aortic insufficiency, conduction defects), and arthritis of proximal joints such as the shoulders and hips.

On a recent visit to New York City, as I was taking a 15-block walk in downtown Manhattan, I was thinking about how fortunate I have been. In 1998 I underwent a transluminal coronary angioplasty with stent placement, and subsequently I received anticoagulant therapy, which resulted in painless hematuria. This led to the discovery of renal-cell carcinoma, for which I had a radical nephrectomy. This experience has prompted me to share with you my perspective as a patient for 44 years, now facing the added uncertainty that a cancer patient has to live with.

You see, I have had arthritis since age 12, and my physician at the time, the chief of orthopedic surgery at the local university hospital, treated me with frequent bed rests and hospitalizations. There were no rheumatologists in Pakistan in those days. He, at one point, prescribed one full year of antituberculous treatment (streptomycin injections, isoniazid, and para-aminosalicylic acid), without any resultant clinical benefit. Later on, he treated me intravenously with honey imported from West Germany. By then I was 16 years old and had just become a medical student.

Two years later, during my first clinical rotation in medical school, I spoke to my teacher, a professor in the department of medicine, about my symptoms. He examined me and diagnosed my disease as ankylosing spondylitis. It primarily involved my back, hip joints, and, to a lesser extent, my neck and shoulders. He prescribed phenylbutazone, a nonsteroidal anti-inflammatory drug, to relieve my pain and stiffness, and it worked effectively.

Soon after I graduated from medical school in 1965, when I was 21, Pakistan was attacked by its neighbor, and I decided to enlist in the Pakistan Army Medical Corps. In my zeal to serve the nation in its hour of need—a nation that had accepted me as a 3-year-old refugee and had provided me with almost free medical education—I did not reveal my illness. My service in the Pakistani Armed Forces was a great experience.

In 1967, when I had just left the army, I received a call for assistance from the very professor from medical school who had diagnosed my ankylosing spondylitis. This professor wanted me to treat his best friend, a prominent local businessman, who had just experienced an acute myocardial infarction. I provided the necessary care, including, later that day, successfully resuscitating the patient when he experienced cardiac arrest. (He would go on to live for another 28 years and help build a hospital for the needy, but that is another story entirely.)

I arrived in London in the summer of 1967 to begin my postgraduate medical studies—despite my arthritis, which never ceased to plague me—in an effort to pursue my goal of an academic career in medicine. Cardiology was my initial choice for a medical subspecialty, but I felt that the anticipated decrease of my spinal mobility, as well as having limited chest expansion due to my ankylosing spondylitis, might one day impair my ability to resuscitate patients. During the required one year of residency training, I chose orthopedics as my surgical elective. While assisting the surgeons in various orthopedic procedures, including total hip arthroplasty, I was keenly aware that the tables would someday be turned and I would be the one at the receiving end of the operation.

I came to the United States in the summer of 1969 and have successfully pursued an academic career in rheumatology. Knowing what it feels like to be an arthritis sufferer, and therefore having a special empathy for patients with this condition, my choice of subspecialty was an easy one to make.

Not surprisingly, my primary research interests have included ankylosing spondylitis and related spondyloarthropathies, along with the associated genetic marker HLA-B27.

Inevitably, the tables did turn, and I experienced the following: bilateral total hip joint replacement; revision hip arthroplasty; fracture of the cervical spine; nonunion of the fracture and another three months of immobilization; recurrent episodes of acute anterior uveitis; hypertension and coronary artery disease; coronary transluminal balloon angioplasties on three separate occasions; and most recently, right radical nephrectomy. Perhaps you will agree that my many encounters as a patient serve as sufficient "qualification," if we can call them that, to assert my own viewpoint. I am very grateful to modern medicine for keeping me going. In some ways, I consider myself a "bionic man." My ankylosing spondylitis, however, has resulted in a complete fusion of my whole spine, including the neck. I cannot turn or even nod my head, and I have to bend at my hip joints to give an impression of a nod. I need to grab onto something to pull myself up from a squatting position. I have virtually no chest expansion. One can imagine what might happen to me if I were to have the misfortune of being in an accident or needing cardiac resuscitation; the probability would be high that, inadvertently, my death would be hastened because of a possible neck fracture or broken ribs.

Although I have always sought the best care possible for myself, I have been unlucky on many occasions in not receiving optimum medical care. However, being a perpetual optimist, I am thankful that I am still alive. I sometimes like to give the analogy of the old Timex watch commercial, because I keep on ticking. But if my personal experiences as a patient were extrapolated to the population at large, they would unfortunately highlight many deficiencies in the current practices of medicine, even here in the United States: the unreceptive receptionists, the allied health professionals who lack empathy for their "clients," and the physicians for whom time is such a precious commodity that they start looking at their wristwatches just minutes into the history-taking to signal their impatience.

We physicians frequently do not acquire the skills of a good communicator, and we often neglect patient education. The word "doctor," as I understand it, means an educator or communicator. Yet some physicians apparently lack the traits required to be a good communicator, and some claim they simply have no time for it anyway. In such situations, an allied health professional, such as a nurse practitioner, could better handle communication with the patients. Better physician-patient communication is certainly needed.

I underwent bilateral hip arthroplasty as a single surgical procedure at a hospital that specialized in such surgeries. A few years later, I had to undergo a revision hip arthroplasty. Before I left the hospital, I noticed that one leg was now shorter than the other by about a half-inch, but my surgeon would not acknowledge this. I still, to this day, wear a shoe lift to minimize my limp.

My first transluminal coronary angioplasty resulted in an extensive internal tear. When I subsequently had restenosis of the involved artery, I was advised by an independent consultant to have a stent inserted at the time of the revision angioplasty. I had my second angioplasty performed at a highly rated medical center and, although I had requested a stent placement, none was given, and my angina symptoms recurred shortly thereafter.

When I fractured my neck, I was treated with the placement of a halo and a vest to immobilize the fracture. I pointed out to my surgeon on numerous occasions that the fracture was not fully immobilized, as was most noticeable when I leaned back or tried to lie on my back. I voiced my concern that the back plate of the vest was not properly conforming to my thoracic kyphosis, but the surgeon repeatedly reassured me that everything was fine. I had to sleep sitting upright. After three months, a radiograph revealed nonunion of the fracture. Subsequently, the vest was changed, but precious time had already been wasted; because months of further immobilization did not heal the fracture, I ultimately needed a surgical fusion.

I have never sued anyone. My forgiving and nonlitigious nature tells me that as patients we should always give our physicians the benefit of the doubt, just as we physicians, likewise, should always show respect for our patients and give them some degree of latitude. But in our current healthcare system, there is an obvious need for a more open dialogue between physicians and their patients.

During the seven-month period in which I wore a halo that was screwed into my skull and attached to a vest that surrounded my chest (just imagine trying to sleep at night wearing all that hardware!) I continued to care for my patients. I found myself in ever greater awe at the power we, as physicians, hold as healers. On one occasion, a new patient came to see me, and after our initial handshake, I noticed that his face was turning pale. I immediately had him lie down on the examination table just before he fainted. When he felt better, the patient started to laugh, and said, "Doc, I had been hurting and waiting to see you for two weeks, but with one look at you, all pains are gone!"

One morning, a few days later, I was walking by the emergency room on my way to the office and had not yet donned my white coat. A young child noticed my halo and asked, "What happened?"

"I had an accident," I replied.

Having surmised that I was en route to the emergency room for acute medical attention, the child inquired, "Is that the steering wheel of your car that is stuck around your head?"

I have enjoyed every bit of my life, with all its humor, hardships, hurdles, and dramatics that could even appeal to the Hollywood movie moguls. And I continue to enjoy my walks. After all, my doctor has instructed me to get daily exercise.

Pablo Casal

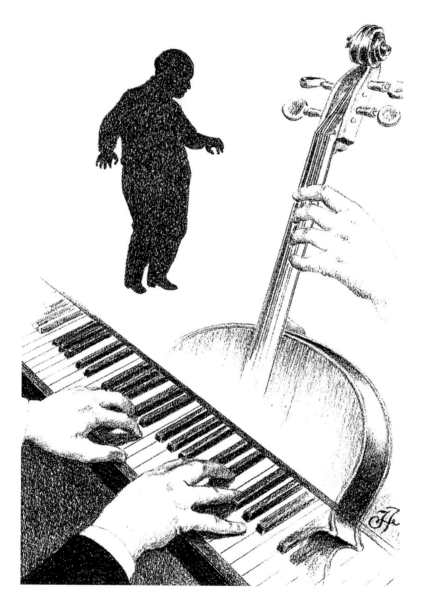

Illustrated by Herb Packard

Pablo Casals was a superb Spanish cellist, composer, and conductor.

Anatomy of an Illness

By Norman Cousins

Norman Cousins was a well-known author, editor of the Saturday Review, and a lecturer at the U.C.L.A. School of Medicine. His successful struggle against a crippling illness is described in his book Anatomy of an Illness. *Even though he was not a physician, his ideas are widely respected by the medical profession. In Rene Dubos' introduction to Cousins' book, he states, 'The basic theme is that every person must accept a certain measure of responsibility for his or her recovery from disease or disability whenever possible." This book shows that our minds can help protective mechanisms in the body combat disease, that "laughter, courage, and tenacity" should be encouraged by patients and caregivers. Norman Cousins also describes the miraculous effect of music on the life of Pablo Casals.*

This book is about a serious illness that occurred in 1964. I was reluctant to write about it for many years because I was fearful of creating false hope in others who were similarly afflicted. Moreover, I knew that a single case has small standing in the annals of medical research, having little more than "anecdotal" or "testimonial" value. However, references to the illness surfaced from time to time in the general and medical press. People wrote to ask whether it was true that I "laughed" my way out of a crippling disease that doctors believed to be irreversible. In view of those questions, I thought it useful to provide a fuller account than appeared in those early reports.

In August 1964, I flew home from a trip abroad with a slight fever. The malaise, which took the form of a generalized feeling of achiness, rapidly deepened. Within a week it became difficult to move my neck, arms, hands, fingers, and legs. My sedimentation rate was over 80. Of all the diagnostic tests, the "sed" rate is one of the most useful to the physician. The way it works is beautifully simple. The speed with which red cells settle in a test tube—measured in millimeters per hour—is generally proportionate to the severity of an inflammation or infection. A normal illness, such as grippe, might produce a sedimentation rate of, say, 30 or even 40. When the rate goes well beyond 60 or 70, however, the physician knows that he is dealing with more than a casual problem. I was hospitalized when the sed rate hit 88. Within a week it was up to 115, generally considered to be a sign of a critical condition.

Cousins' personal physician was very candid with him about his case.

He reviewed the reports of the various specialists he had called in as consultants. He said there was no agreement on a precise diagnosis. There was, however, a consensus that I was suffering from a serious collagen illness—a disease of the connective tissue. All arthritic and rheumatic diseases are in this category. Collagen is the fibrous substance that binds the cells together. In a sense then, I was coming unstuck. I had considerable difficulty in moving my limbs and even in turning over in bed. Nodules appeared on my body—gravel-like substances under the skin—indicating the systemic nature of the disease. At the low point of my illness, my jaws were almost locked.

Experts from Howard Rusk's rehabilitation clinic in New York confirmed the presence of collagen disease, adding the more specific diagnosis of ankylosing spondylitis that causes degeneration of the spine. He was told that full recovery was unlikely.

I must not make it appear that all my infirmities disappeared overnight. For many months I couldn't get my arms up far enough to reach for a book on a high shelf. My fingers weren't agile enough to do what I wanted them to do on the organ keyboard. My neck had a limited turning radius. My knees were somewhat wobbly, and off and on, I have had to wear a metal brace. Even so, I was sufficiently recovered to go back to my job at the *Saturday Review* full-time again, and this was miracle enough for me.

Is the recovery a total one? Year by year the mobility has improved. I have become pain free, except for my shoulder and knees, although I have been able to discard the metal braces. I no longer feel a sharp twinge in my wrists when I hit a tennis ball or golf ball as I did for a long time. I can ride a horse flat out and hold a camera with a steady hand. And I have recaptured my ambition to play the Toccata and Fugue in D-Minor, though I find the going slower and tougher than I had hoped. My neck has a full turning radius again, despite the statement by specialists as recently as 1971 that the condition was degenerative and that I would have to adjust to a quarter turn.

People have asked what I thought when I was told by the specialists that my disease was progressive and incurable. The answer is simple. Since I didn't accept the verdict, I wasn't trapped in a cycle of fear, depression, and panic that frequently accompanies a supposedly incurable illness. I must not make it seem, however, that I was not unmindful of the seriousness of the problem or that I was in a festive mood throughout. Being unable to move my body was all the evidence I needed that the specialists were dealing with real concerns. But deep down, I knew I had a good chance and relished the idea of bucking the odds.

Pablo Casals' Influence on Cousins' Life

The following observations about Pablo Casals by Norman Cousins reveal the astonishing impact of music on Don Pablo's energy and will to live. Don Pablo was a Spanish cellist and one of the greatest musicians of his time.

I met him for the first time at his home in Puerto Rico just a few weeks before his ninetieth birthday. I was fascinated by his daily routine. About 8 a.m., his lovely young wife Marta would help him to start the day. His various infirmities made it difficult for him to dress himself. Judging from his difficulty in walking and from the way he held his arms, I guessed he was suffering from rheumatoid arthritis. His emphysema was evident in his labored breathing. He came into the living room on Marta's arm. He was badly stooped. His head was pitched forward and he walked with a shuffle. His hands were swollen and his fingers were clenched.

Even before going to the breakfast table, Don Pablo went to the piano—which I learned was a daily ritual. He arranged himself with some difficulty on the piano bench; then, with discernible effort, raised his swollen and clenched fingers above the keyboard.

I was not prepared for the miracle that was about to happen. The fingers slowly unlocked and reached toward the keys like the buds of a plant toward the sunlight. His back straightened. He seemed to breathe more freely. Now his fingers settled on the keys. Then came the opening bars of Bach's Wohtemperierte Klavier, played with great sensitivity and control. I had forgotten that Don Pablo had achieved proficiency on several musical instruments before he took up the cello. He hummed as he played. Then said that Bach spoke to him here—and he placed his hand over his heart.

Then he plunged into a Brahms concerto and his fingers, now agile and powerful, raced across the keyboard with dazzling speed. His entire body seemed fused with the music. It was no longer stiff and shrunken, but supple and graceful and completely free of its arthritic coils.

Having finished the piece, he stood up by himself, far straighter and taller than when he had come into the room. He walked to the breakfast table with no trace of a shuffle, ate heartily, talked animatedly, finished the meal, and went for a walk on the beach.

After an hour or so, he came back to the house and napped. When he rose, the stoop and the shuffle and the clenched hands were back again. On this particular day, a camera and recording crew from public television was scheduled to arrive in mid-afternoon. Anticipating the visit, Don Pablo said he wished some way could be found to call it off; he didn't feel up to the exertion of the filming, with its innumerable and inexplicable retakes and the extreme heat of the bright lights.

Marta, having been through these reluctances before, reassured Don Pablo, saying she was certain he would be stimulated by the meeting. She reminded him that he liked the young people who did the last filming and that they would probably be back again. In particular, she called his attention to the lovely young lady who directed the recording. Don Pablo brightened. "Yes, of course," he said. "It will be good to see them again."

As before, he stretched his arms in front of him and extended his fingers. Then the spine straightened and he stood up and went to his cello. He began to play. His fingers, hands, and arms were in sublime coordination as they responded to the demands of his brain for the controlled beauty of movement and tone. Any cellist thirty years his junior would have been proud to have such extraordinary physical command.

Twice in one day I had seen the miracle. A man almost ninety, beset with the infirmities of old age, was able to cast off his afflictions, at least temporarily, because he knew he had something of overriding importance to do. There is no mystery about the way it worked, for it happened every day. Creativity for Pablo Casals was the source of his own cortisone. It is doubtful whether any anti-inflammatory medication he would have taken would have been as powerful or as safe as the substances produced by the interaction of his mind and body.

Count Leo Tolstoy

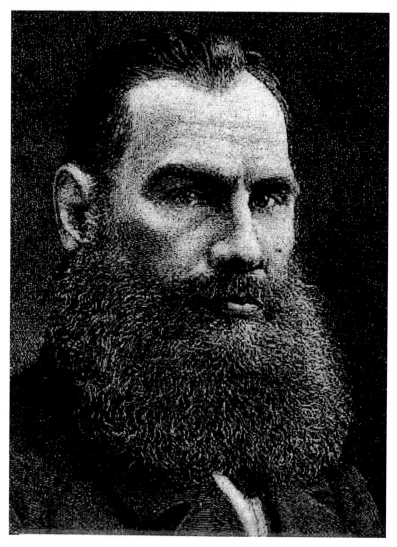

Photo of Leo Tolstoy (approximately 1863)

Finding Hope & Compassion

The Old Grandfather and the Grandson

By Leo Tolstoy
with Commentary by Robert Coles, M.D.

Robert Coles, who is a professor of psychiatry and medical humanities at Harvard Medical School, is also James Agee Professor of Social Ethics at Harvard. In his book The Moral Intelligence of Children, *he describes the responses of teachers and children to Leo Tolstoy's story, "The Old Grandfather and the Grandson," that stir up lively discussions about moral values and compassion.*

The Russian writer Tolstoy, who lived from 1828 to 1910, was one of the greatest novelists and storytellers in world literature. His compelling story tells how two parents learned about compassion from their own young son. Seeing his grandfather being neglected in his own home, this boy did not want the same thing to happen to his parents.

The grandfather had become very old. His legs wouldn't go, his eyes didn't see, his ears didn't hear, he had no teeth. And when he ate, the food dripped from his mouth. The son and daughter-in-law stopped setting a place for him at the table and gave him supper in back of the stove. Once they brought dinner down to him in a cup. The old man wanted to move the cup and dropped and broke it. The daughter-in-law began to grumble at the old man for spoiling everything in the house and breaking the cups and said that she would now give him dinner in a dishpan. The old man only sighed and said nothing.

Once the husband and wife were staying at home and watching their small son playing on the floor with some wooden planks; he was building something. The father asked. "What is that you are doing, Misha?" And Misha said: "Dear Father, I am making a dishpan. So that when you and dear Mother become old, you may be fed from this dishpan." The husband and wife looked at one another and began to weep. They became ashamed of so offending the old man, and from then on seated him at the table and waited on him.

Commentary by Robert Coles

I've used that Tolstoy story with various kinds of students. I've read it aloud. I've asked for interpretations of it, comments about it, thoughts about what it has to say to us. I've told the class how I got to know the story, from my mother's love of Tolstoy; I told of her reading his various stories and novels over and over again, of her habit of reading them aloud to my father.

I've told the class of certain events in my life, times when I've failed to respond to that story, failed to respond to this person or that person, so preoccupied was I with my own responsibilities and interests. The point of such personal stories, I say, is not self-accusation, nor am I ironically intent on getting myself off a hook by publicly putting myself on it, in the hope that the students will soothe my soul. The point is to summon one's frail side so as to enable a more forthright sharing of experiences on the part of all of us; that guy has stumbled, and he's not making too much of it, but he *is* putting it on the table, and thereby I'm enabled to put some of myself, my remembrances, my story, on the table, whether explicitly, by speaking up or, in the way many of us do, by also remembering—another's memories trigger our own. In time, after we've talked, I've asked the students to write an essay about the Tolstoy story, about its meaning to them, about what they imagine themselves doing with the story if they were parents or teachers. Soon enough, of course, I am reading introspective memoirs or suggestions for this or that course of action—all of us become witnesses, with Tolstoy's help, to the moral imagination at work.

For years, as a volunteer teacher in an elementary school, I have used the Tolstoy story, and witnessed firsthand a moral fable's magical power to prompt a young reader's empathic response. Some of those readers (charmingly, instructively, poignantly) want us all to take Tolstoy's story to heart by literally living it out: "We could be told to eat in some corner, out of a dishpan, and, wow, we'd sure remember what that was like," so a girl of ten insisted.

A boy of nine was more elaborate: "Half of us would eat at a table and there would be a tablecloth, and the nice dishes, and half would be on the floor, in the corners, or someplace with the dishpan. Then we could all switch—and then we would know." "What would we know?" the eager teacher asks. "We'd know what it feels like the one way, and then the other," the wide-eyed boy, filled with a kind of adventurous enthusiasm, replied.

A girl has her version of a kind of moral theater: "We could throw dice or something, so if you have bad luck, you'll get the dishpan treatment. Then you'll really feel sorry for yourself, and you won't just forget." She seems finished with her scenario—only to add this: "We should try to help the person with the dishpan. I mean, if I was on the floor, and I was getting my food that way, and it wasn't as good, the food, as the food others were getting, eating in good dishes at a table, and then someone came over, and she offered to give me a better dish, or better food, and told me I could stand up and sit with the rest of the people at the dining room table—then I'd sure be grateful to that person, and if I saw someone else sitting over there on the floor, in the corner, and they (he or she) was eating bread and water, like that, from a dishpan, then I'd want to go and help them, I know I would; I'd want to invite them over and give them a nice dish, because if you have been there, in trouble, you'll know, you'll remember, and you'll want to help the next guy who's there, I think."

A more skeptical girl, also nine, wasn't, alas, so sure that such would inevitably be the case—and did *she* get us all going: a real gift. "How do you know," she wondered aloud, "if someone would remember the dishpan a year later?" We didn't "know," of course—but she continued her inquiry, expanded it in this manner: "What if someone got really mad sitting on the floor, and she said to herself, I'm here, now, eating out of the dishpan, but if I get lucky and I get out of this, or if I work my way out of it—if somehow this ends, what's happened to me, then I'll get even with the people, because they did this to me. I'll make *them* eat out of the dishpan, or I'll just try to forget all this! I'll say, don't remind me of all my troubles; they're gone! Couldn't that be the way, the way it could work out?"

To play that portion of a tape-recorded class discussion is to bring to the listener a reminder: the variousness of our possible responses to an affecting, compelling, moral fable, the work of a master, a giant among writers. That girl just quoted was quite in touch with her own family's world, as she lets us know with this terse, final comment: "My father says it's best to forget pain, once it's over." The children nod readily—and why not? "Who wants to hold on to pain?" another girl asked, asserted, seconded. Nor was I quick to take exception. A long spell of quiet, however, gave me time to think—and think and think: How to get us into a kind of reflection that would bring us back to the Tolstoyan spirit we'd initially embraced upon reading his short, morally evocative story. My eventual comment: "One way, I guess, to deal with pain is to try to learn how to spare others what you've gone through yourself."

How to justify, actually, my saying more—a continued effort to steer this moral discussion in a direction that pleases me? A rescue—a girl who raises her hand and speaks simultaneously before I have a chance to recognize her: "Pain is no good, but sometimes it just has to happen." Why? An immediate rejoinder: "Because," the girl replies—but no follow-up, and I feel dejected, tempted to give a disquisition tailored to the age of my class. I'm still not able to accept the moral vitality of these children, their willingness, their capacity to delve into the very matters Tolstoy has explored—and expressly for fellow human beings of their age, no less! Again a deliverance, from another girl: "Because—because that's what it's like sometimes." "What do you mean, what are you talking about?" The boy is relentless, I think—He'll be a lawyer, a prosecuting attorney one day. But the girl is undeterred, unfazed, quite sure of herself. "See, there are times when it's true—'no pain, no gain'—that's what my dad says. My mom—she told me you can't be born without your mother being in pain."

While that pointed example settles in, I feel pleased, and suddenly, quite admiring of this class, its moral possibilities, capability.

I look at the clock—just a few minutes before the bell tells us to stop. As the children explode into recess noise, I wonder what our intense discussion will mean to them, if anything, a few hours hence, never mind a week or two down the line.

Henry James' nephew, the son of William James, once asked the great and thoughtful novelist what he ought to do with his life, how he ought to live it. The nephew received this advice: "Three things in human life are important. The first is to be kind. The second is to be kind. And the third is to be kind."

Finding Hope & Compassion

The Old Vermonter

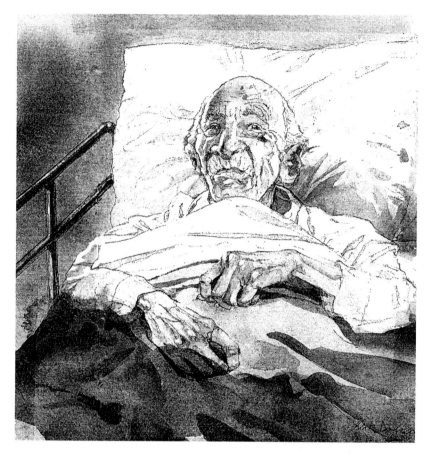

Illustrated by Bert Dodson

The old Vermonter's stoicism made a strong impression on the medical student who was helping to care for him.

One March Morning

By Timothy Rooney, M.D.

The author is a 2001 graduate of Dartmouth Medical School and a 1987 graduate of Dartmouth College. Between completing his undergraduate work and returning to Dartmouth for medical school, he was a pilot for 10 years in the U. S. Navy, flying F-14s from aircraft carriers.

In this article from Dartmouth Medicine, *Dr. Rooney describes an old Vermonter's stoicism that made a strong impression on him when he was a medical student helping to care for the old farmer.*

I saw him in the charcoal half-light of early morning. It was almost dawn on a raw March day, and it was raining in fits and starts. The voices of the nurses were hushed in the semidarkness as they conferred at the end of the night shift. The old man was alone in his curtained-off space, breathing in jerks. I could see his muscles straining underneath his papery skin—the outward signs of an inner struggle.

I had first met him just three weeks before, as a third-year medical student on one of the surgery teams. Internal medicine had asked surgery to consult on an inpatient, and I had offered to go along to help the surgical resident.

We found this 93-year-old Vermonter lying rigid in his hospital bed. As he tried to answer our questions, we could see and feel his taut abdominal muscles standing guard of their own accord, hiding the tender structures beneath. He whispered to us in between bouts of pain, telling us that until a few days before he had been living alone on his farm. The sudden and intense crampiness that we were watching had brought him reluctantly first to his doctor and then to the hospital.

This story worried the resident, and after a rushed look at the laboratory values and a discussion with the attending surgeon, we decided on immediate surgery. We informed the gaunt gentleman with the searing, glittering eyes of our recommendation, and he uttered what I remember as his only clear, full sentence. He surfaced from the hazy pain for only a moment and told us, "You'll have five days to save me."

Both the resident and I stepped back at this cryptic challenge, wondering at his words and manner. A moment later, we wheeled him upstairs to the operating room, his body cringing with each of the bumps onto the elevator.

I remember my relief as the patient drifted off to the temporary painlessness of anesthesia, but I moved quickly from empathy to curiosity as we scrubbed our hands and prepped his now semirelaxed and pale abdomen. The surgeons quickly opened the layers of skin and fat and muscle and found that the worst had happened. His dark-purple small intestine pushed up through the new wound like a large, grotesque blossom, followed closely by an acrid smell. The loops of his bowel had twisted and died as they had slowly lost blood flow and become more and more inflamed. We could see that the torsion involved almost the entire length of his small intestine.

I alternated between fascination with what I was seeing, nausea from the smell, and wonder at what this might mean for this man. The surgeons told me that while there are a number of causes for a twisted bowel, the only hope for retaining some intestinal function was to remove the dead tissue in an attempt to save the rest. Fortunately, just enough had survived to allow the possibility of normal digestion and absorption. The operation itself went well, and the wound was closed with a long, clean line of staples—a stark contrast to the intruding bulge of moments before.

After the surgery, the old man was kept on the ventilator and rushed to the ICU for postoperative care. We wondered about what sort of stamina might lie dormant in this patient we hardly knew. Would he give up? Or would he fight this thing the way he had fought to live by himself on his farm, well past his 90th birthday, fiercely independent in his private, northern New England way?

Our patient's 85-year-old brother and sister-in-law drove down every few days from northernmost rural Vermont, never quite trusting this strange world of plastic tubing that burrowed under fragile skin. The two of them would come in the ICU together, tears in their eyes, holding hands, and leaning against one another—their rough shoes and flannel shirts contrasting with the shiny, hospital-clean bustle around them. But he told us that he wanted us to take every measure we could to save his older brother.

The irony was that in this most modern unit of modern medicine, we were still waiting for the patient to do the healing. If he could have turned his head just a little and seen through the ointment in his eyes, past the ever-changing numbers on his life-support readout, he might have noticed the delicate, late-March snowflakes that make most of us wonder if spring will ever come. How many times had he chuckled at those same flakes, which seem to mock our optimistic, early shedding of winter coats here in the North Country?

About 10 days after his operation, the patient surprised us all early one morning by coming off the ventilator, short on digestive length but not on fight. He sat up, staring at me and raspingly breathing on his own. It was difficult to meet his gaze. I saw anger and frustration in those eyes. This was a man who would not tolerate life with an ever-present breathing tube.

Was I only imagining it, or was there also a glint in his eyes that said he knew the five days he'd given us had passed almost a week ago? Would he have chosen this course, or had we—with the best of intentions—chipped away at the dignity of this man? And yet, when I saw him on each of the next few mornings, I could picture him back on his land, where he worked vigorously and on his own for so many years.

But soon he took a turn for the worse and had to return to ventilator-assisted breathing. He had aspirated some of the contents of his stomach into his lungs. While we continued to treat him with antibiotics and respiratory support, we were sure that each breath would be his last. His brother eventually, reluctantly, decided on a "do not resuscitate" order.

But a few wet March days later, our patient had battled back yet again and was moved to a ward outside of the intensive care unit.

Very early the next morning, as I stood near the unit's full-length windows and said a prayer to a day just beginning, the old farmer's agonal breaths caught my attention. I wondered if it would be harder for his soul to fly up through the hurrying gray clouds outside, which hid the blue sky and cloaked the early-morning chill. I knew that he would be gone soon, and I prayed for this man whose eyes had spoken to me.

Half an hour later, a nurse came to the edge of our surgical team's tightly clustered circle and told us that the old Vermonter had passed away. I went with the intern to proclaim his death. He looked comfortable lying there, and yet I was sure that I could still see his chest moving. He looked like himself again.

I found the obituary in the paper the day after he died. He had lived in the area his whole life, had worked for the water company, married, raised a son, farmed his land. The newspaper notice also mentioned that he had once dedicated a hydroelectric dam with President Roosevelt, that together they had turned the great, greased handles to open the floodgates.

I never got a chance to ask him what it was like to meet President Roosevelt. But, then again, he would have just waved me away, this solitary Vermont man of actions rather than words.

Kay Redfield Jamison

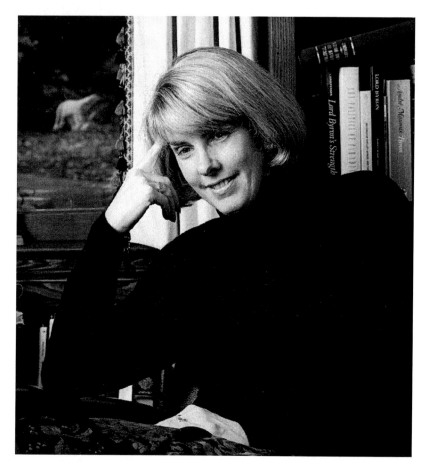

Photo by Tom Wolf

"There is a particular kind of pain, elation, loneliness, and terror involved in this kind of madness."

– Kay Redfield Jamison

A Memoir of Moods and Madness

By Kay Redfield Jamison, Ph.D.

Dr. Jamison is uniquely qualified to describe manic-depressive illness (bipolar disease). She is a professor of psychiatry at the Johns Hopkins University School of Medicine, a therapist, and a survivor of manic-depression herself. Her eloquent description of mood swings that alternate between soaring exaltation and devastating, even suicidal depression help us to understand the intensity of the experience associated with manic-depressive illness. She is the author of the best- selling book An Unquiet Mind, *which discusses manic-depression from her perspective as a patient and a leading authority of this disease.*

Unlike some milder forms of depression, manic-depression causes cyclic upheavals of mania and unexplained depression. A manic phase may produce a very cheerful mood, rapid speech, limitless energy, reckless driving, increased sexual activity, and wild spending sprees with credit cards. The severity and course of manic-depression vary widely in different people. Severe manic-depression can cause psychosis and increase the risk of suicide. During a psychotic episode, an individual is out of touch with reality and may have hallucinations, delusions, or paranoid behavior. Unwillingness to take prescription medication like lithium for control of manic-depression can be catastrophic.

I was a senior in high school when I had my first attack of manic-depressive illness; once the siege began, I lost my mind rather rapidly. At first, everything seemed so easy. I raced about like a crazed weasel, bubbling with plans and enthusiasms, immersed in sports, and staying up all night, night after night, out with friends, reading everything that wasn't nailed down, filling manuscript books with poems and fragments of plays, and making expansive, completely unrealistic, plans for my future. The world was filled with pleasure and promise; I felt great. I felt I could do anything, that no task was too difficult. My mind seemed clear, fabulously focused, and able to make intuitive mathematical leaps that had up to that point eluded me.

I did, finally, slow down. In fact, I came to a grinding halt. Unlike the very severe manic episodes that came a few years later and escalated wildly and psychotically out of control, this first sustained wave of mild mania was a light, lovely tincture of true mania; like hundreds of subsequent periods of high enthusiasms it was short-lived and quickly burned itself out: tiresome to my friends, perhaps; exhausting and exhilarating to me, definitely; but not disturbingly over the top. Then the bottom began to fall out of my life and mind. My thinking, far from being clearer than a crystal, was tortuous. I would read the same passage over and over again only to realize that I had no memory at all for what I had just read. Each book or poem I picked up was the same way. Incomprehensible. Nothing made sense. I would find myself staring out the window with no idea of what was going on around me. It was very frightening.

Now, all of a sudden, my mind had turned on me. It was incapable of concentrated thought and turned time and again to the subject of death: I was going to die.

What difference did anything make? Life's run was only a short and meaningless one, why live? I was totally exhausted and could scarcely pull myself out of bed in the mornings. It took me twice as long to walk anywhere as it ordinarily did, and I wore the same clothes over and over again, as it was otherwise too much of an effort to make a decision about what to put on. I dreaded having to talk with people, avoided my friends whenever possible, and sat in the school library early mornings and late afternoons, virtually inert, with a dead heart and a brain as cold as clay.

I have no idea how I managed to pass as normal in school, except that other people are generally caught up in their own lives and seldom notice despair in others if those despairing make an effort to disguise the pain.

Dr. Jamison describes the depression that follows mania in detail as follows:

It is a pitiless, unrelenting pain that affords no window of hope…There is nothing good to be said for it except it gives you the experience of how it must be to be old and sick and dying; to be slow of mind; to have no belief in the possibilities of life, the pleasures of sex, the exquisiteness of music, or the ability to make yourself and others laugh. It is flat, hollow, tiresome and unendurable; a gray, bleak preoccupation with death, dying and decay.

There is a particular kind of pain, elation, loneliness, and terror involved in this kind of madness. When you're high it's tremendous. The ideas and feelings are fast and frequent like shooting stars, and you follow them until you find better and brighter ones. Shyness goes, the right words and gestures are suddenly there, the power to captivate others a felt certainty. There are interests found in uninteresting people. Sensuality is pervasive and the desire to seduce and be seduced irresistible. Feelings of ease, intensity, well-being, financial omnipotence, and euphoria pervade one's

Finding Hope & Compassion

marrow. But, somewhere, this changes. The fast ideas are far too fast, and there are far too many; overwhelming confusion replaces clarity. Memory goes. Humor and absorption on friends' faces are replaced by fear and concern. Everything previously moving with the grain is now against—you are irritable, angry, frightened, uncontrollable, and enmeshed totally in the blackest caves of the mind. You never knew those caves were there. It will never end, for madness carries its own reality.

I have often asked myself whether, given the choice, I would choose to have manic-depressive illness. If lithium were not available to me, or didn't work for me, the answer would be a simple no—and it would be an answer laced with terror. But lithium does work for me, and therefore, I suppose I can afford to pose the question. Strangely enough I think I would choose to have it. It's complicated. Depression is awful beyond words or sounds or images; I would not go through an extended one again. It bleeds relationships through suspicion, lack of confidence and self-respect, the inability to enjoy life, to walk or talk or think normally, the exhaustion, the night terrors, the day terrors.

People cannot abide being around you when you are depressed. They think that they ought to, and they might even try, but you know and they know that you are tedious beyond belief: You're irritable and paranoid and humorless and lifeless and critical and demanding and no reassurance is enough. You're frightened, and you're frightening, and you're 'not at all like yourself but will be soon,' but you know you won't.

So why would I want anything to do with this illness? Because I honestly believe as a result of it I have felt more things, more deeply; had more experiences, more intensely; loved more, and been more loved; laughed more often for having cried more often; appreciated more the springs, for all the winters; worn death "as close as dungarees," appreciated it—and life—more; seen the finest and the most terrible in people, and slowly learned the values of caring, loyalty and seeing things through. I have seen the breadth and depth and width of my mind and heart and seen how frail they both are, and how ultimately unknowable they both are. Depressed, I have crawled on my hands and knees in order to get across a room and have done it for month after month. But normal or manic, I have run faster, thought faster, and loved faster than most I know. And I think much of this is related to my illness—the intensity it gives to things and the perspective it forces on me. I think it has made me test the limits of my mind and the limits of my upbringing, family education, and friends.

"I doubt sometimes whether a quiet and unagitated life would have suited me—yet I sometimes long for it."

—Lord Byron

Anne Foley

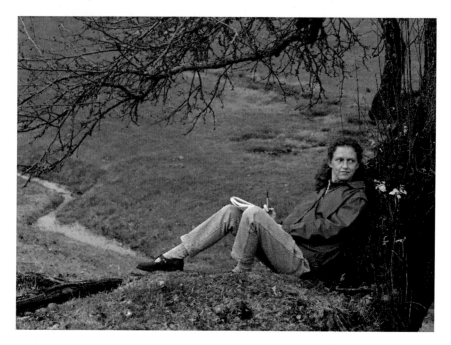

Photo by Jon Gilbert Fox

Anne Foley drew on her journal entries over the past two years to write this article. She often chooses outdoor settings like this one to write in her journal.

Regaining What's Been Lost

By Anne Foley
Introduction by Lee McDavid

The article by Anne Foley that follows was published in Dartmouth Medi-cine, *Winter 2001. Lee McDavid, who wrote the introductory commentary under the title, "Only clad with skin," is a freelance writer and regular contributor to* Dartmouth Medicine.

Anne Foley has anorexia nervosa, which is a severe and sometimes fatal eating disorder that amounts to self-starvation. It is often considered a consequence of our modern society's obsession with thinness, yet as long ago as 1689 an English physician described the syndrome as "a skeleton only clad with skin."

Today, the American Psychiatric Association recognizes two specific categories of eating disorders: anorexia nervosa and bulimia nervosa. Both are characterized by a preoccupation with body weight and shape. In the case of anorexia, affected individuals— most commonly adolescent females—have an intense fear of gaining weight or becoming fat, despite a weight that is less than 85 percent of what is considered normal for their age and height. What may start as a simple diet—possibly after a suggestion by a teacher, coach, or parent to lose a few pounds—turns into an increasingly restrictive eating regi-men. Excessive exercise and purging (self-induced vomiting or abuse of laxatives or diu-retics) may accompany the starvation diet. But even when anorexics have become emaci-ated, they look in the mirror and see only fat.

The term "anorexia," which means "loss of appetite," is actually a misnomer. People with anorexia are preoccupied with food, but they deny their need to eat. Their ability to abstain from food often makes them feel proud of their self-control, but it also creates overwhelming feelings of guilt and shame.

While anorexics seek weight loss primarily by restricting how much they eat, bulimia nervosa is characterized by binge eating—consuming large amounts of food in a short period of time—followed by purging. Although some anorexics also engage in binge-purge behavior, the anorexic loses weight while the bulimic usually hovers around normal weight.

The National Association of Anorexia Nervosa and Associated Diseases es-timates that, in this country, seven million women and one million men suffer from eating disorders. Bulimia is more prevalent than anorexia among males; 95 percent of anorexics are female, and most are adolescents and young adults. As many as one percent of high school and college-age women may have anorexia nervosa, and four percent may have bulimia nervosa.

The physiological and psychological consequences of anorexia are devastating; they include depression, social withdrawal, and insomnia, as well as heart, kidney, and liver damage—and even death. And recovery can be a long, slow process.

Dr. Richard Ferrell was the director of Dartmouth-Hitchcock Medical Center Inpatient psychiatry service in 1983 when he first met with Anne Foley and diagnosed her as having anorexia. "Despite much effort," he explains, "researchers have found no firm answers as to the cause of anorexia. Early family experiences, social pressures, the desire to delay sexual maturity, genetics, and mineral deficiencies have all been suggested. The most honest thing to say about causation is that the cause is truly unknown," Ferrell admits.

"What is known is the importance of family and friends in the recognition of anorexia. Often a family member is the first person to notice an anorexic's severe weight loss and to encourage the individual to seek help. Anorexics typically rebuff efforts to alter their behavior, but once in psychotherapy, they can begin to recover.

"My role is to listen, first and foremost," explains Ferrell, who has been on the Dartmouth Medical School faculty since 1975 and is now associate professor of psychiatry. "It's also to try to correct misperceptions that a patient has about him or herself. Building a realistic self-image and working toward greater self-esteem are the primary components of helping a person with anorexia."

The following article is adapted from Anne Foley's journal entries over many years.

Regaining What's Been Lost

I have not been living with grace in my body, because an illness binds me up. For 20 years I have been unhappy and working hard to break from my confinement. Misery was my motivation, but hope is what directs my steps. Hope and progress go hand in hand—my hope for a fuller life fuels my progress, and steps of progress fuel my hope.

If my illness were a physical ailment, such as cancer, I would be broadcasting my recovery for all to hear. I would be advertising my strides toward health by dancing in the streets. But the illness I have is labeled a mental illness. And who dares to talk about such a thing? My long ordeal is covered up as though it never happened, whereas the truth is that it has shaped my life.

Why do I hang my head in shame over an illness I never chose to have? It crept in on me. It wove its nasty tentacles into me and stole away parts of my life. Somehow, I had the feeling I was being cradled even when it should have been obvious I was being strangled. The monster caused me to be blind, until eventually I was stumbling about, struggling, growing so very tired. It took some time in hospitals, plus a fine psychiatrist, to loosen the monster's grip. Now I am learning to walk again. When I can hold my head up and step lightly, I will dance.

My doctor's role in my recovering has been immeasurable, and I thank God for my good fortune in finding him. He has a very difficult job, and he does it with patience. No drugs can be prescribed to cure my diseased cells. No pages in a textbook will give step-by-step instructions for a remedy. Rather, the doctor's role is similar to that of an artist who is helping me to paint a picture of a life of health and freedom. He points my head in the right direction, and with persistence, he describes what this picture might look like.

Many people die from this illness, but even though I recognize that danger, I play with it like I'm running along the edge of a cliff. I dodge left and right among rocks that might trip me and send me over the edge, but the risk is exciting. Maybe without the cliff's edge as a landmark, I would be lost. Maybe I need it as a trail marker. But there might be another way.

The Label

This mental illness that I struggle against has the label of "anorexia nervosa." Having a name for my troubles helps me to understand that I am not at fault here, nor am I some kind of mutant. To be able to think of my malady as an illness rather than a choice frees me from the guilt of feeling like a bad person who makes bad decisions.

The most concern has always been my weight. This red flag may have been a saving grace, as it was the only cry for help I was able to make at times. I was not able to tell anyone how I was suffering. But like a high fever, my sudden loss of weight alerted those around me to my inner troubles. Unfortunately, however, more problems developed when people tried to help me by concentrating on how many pounds I gained or lost. I felt reduced to a number, and frustration mounted on all sides when I couldn't respond to kindly offered and seemingly simple solutions. If I would just put butter on my toast. Drink whole milk. Have some pizza with everyone else. Just eat—damn it! I had always believed myself to be a good girl, and I wanted to be a good girl still. So I began to lie. "Yes, I ate breakfast." "No, I didn't drink water before being weighed." I became a master: watering down soups and smoothies that were prepared for me, slipping bread into my pockets and slices of cheese between the pages of books I read at mealtime.

Yet lying made me bad. And I knew that sooner or later I would be found out. This is one way I lost self-respect, and on its heels came a growing self-hatred. Soon enough I had a screaming voice inside me telling me I was absolutely no good. Any help would be wasted on me. Couldn't they all see how awful I was? Death, I thought at times, was the only way out.

Once I was able to accept that my suffering had a label and that I was not alone in these struggles, I could reach out for professional help. I found a far-sighted doctor who could see me as a person. He had studied eating disorders but did not claim to know all about me. I certainly share characteristics with other anorexics, but it's been critical that I feel recognized and valued as an individual.

Unsure of myself though I may be, this doctor listens to me patiently. Despite the fact that I am often ashamed of myself and hesitant to reveal myself, he waits quietly as little by little I test his tolerance of me. He has never reacted negatively. I then find the courage to go on and reveal more. I discover aspects of myself that have long been buried beneath symptoms.

I am now realizing that I have lost a lot during the long course of this illness. The lost pounds are only the most tangible sign of the losses. But it's hard to get a firm grasp on things when the ground beneath me is still shifting. Slowly I am finding my balance and standing taller, with more assurance. Now I can see more frequently and clearly the things that I lost, and I want them back.

Emotions

Like many others, I fell into anorexia at a time when I was vulnerable. I was adolescent, feeling my way into adulthood and putting on a show to mask all my insecurities. I was extremely confused as I left the familiarity of my home and family for the first time and headed off to college.

My parents had recently separated and were going through a divorce. The first big loss was the security of solid love at home. The family I had banked on was in collapse, yet home was like a tether on my legs. I wanted to leave it, to stretch my wings, but flap as I might, I didn't have the strength to pull away.

I am now learning that perfect love—something I dreamed a cohesive family represented—doesn't exist. And I am learning that there is nothing inherently wrong with me, that I don't repel all love. I may still be disappointed, and I may disappoint, but no one is perfect. Corrections can be made.

I must watch my every step, because at any time I could topple from the cliff that my illness pulls me toward. Yet as my physical health has improved with weight gain, I am still walking further from the cliff's edge. My footing isn't quite so critical. I can take my eyes off my feet now and look up. I can enjoy the moment—soak in life. I can smile and even laugh. I can make others laugh. I have found humor again!

In many ways, anorexia made my world shrink. As my body became smaller, so did my emotional environment. I folded in on myself and crawled into a cave. Maybe I could harden myself so nothing could hurt me. A close friend began to call me "Rocky." I focused on little else besides what I would or would not eat, had or had not eaten. On how to avoid being in social situations that might possibly involve a meal.

In hindsight, I believe that the starved body causes much of this shutdown. Though I lived in the midst of plenty, my life felt like a barren crater on the side of a beautifully forested mountain. I could hide out in such a place.

As I take steps out of my cave, I notice more of my surroundings. I can now pay attention to a wider variety of things. I recall taking a walk with a friend one noontime—asking questions about her life and really listening to her replies. My mind wasn't funneled entirely toward what to do about lunch. After she left I felt so good that I had finally been able to give all my attention to someone. This happens more often now.

As the years passed, it became difficult to remember a life without the dictates of my illness. When I first began to laugh again, my cheeks hurt. When I gain even a couple of pounds, I feel bloated and big. When I indulge in some self-gratifying purchase, I feel selfish and wasteful. Slowly I am repeating these behaviors; practice brings some ease, and I am loosening up, breaking free. Every time I peek out of the anorexic cave, I can see what a dull and stale place it is.

Anorexia is like a cruel dictator from whom I've had to free myself—an all-powerful inner voice that kept screaming at me to do this or that. I accepted this voice and let it rule me. Never has it been kind to me. It puts me down in the worst possible way and holds me there. Yet I have let myself believe that it is protecting me. The hardest part of recovery has been getting this screaming voice to move out.

With growing freedom comes flexibility. Anorexia is very stiff, with a flat expression and a monotonal voice. Rigid. Colorless. As I recover, I am regaining the ability to bend and move freely. Not everything has to be absolute. I can yield. I can look at issues from a variety of angles. There is a slackening of the rules I live under. A world that once looked black and white takes on color. This is terrifying, except that it is happening gradually and I have learned to adjust.

I am starting to believe that there is something about low body weight that instigates rigor. I was not so stiff before losing weight. I did behave by a set of standards, trying to be a "good girl," but within those boundaries I moved about freely. There was joy and fullness, color, and life. I laughed. I was spontaneous. I pitched a fast softball and was graceful on the ski slopes. I was healthy. I ate.

When I stopped eating enough, my body shut down. My mind also shut down. As I weakened, I felt powerless to push back against that which was suffocating me.

Initially, I lost weight because I became upset and depressed and lost my appetite. Being a freshman in college at the time, I was surrounded by the usual female malady of concern over weight and body size. I attracted attention and even praise as my weight dropped, and other women frequently commented in the dining hall that they wished they had my willpower.

When a friend was looking for a running companion, I joined her for early morning jogs. When rain, snow, sleet, cramps, or term papers detained her, I went by myself. Soon enough I had crossed the border from thin to sick, but it was others who recognized this, not me.

By then I had established a list of what I could and could not eat. Rules. I frequently broke the rules, which brought guilt and then punishment, which resulted in more weight loss. I was caught in a tangle of appetite and restrictions—guilty in my court if I ate, guilty in other's court if I didn't. There was no way to win as long as I reduced my self-worth to controlling my most basic bodily needs.

Appetites

I gradually lost many appetites during my years with this illness. The first was the appetite for food and the pleasures of eating. I began to appreciate a growling stomach as I lay in bed at night. The hunger that I did not let myself alleviate served as a reminder that there was a world of good things around me that I was not worthy of. I gave food great power.

I decided early on to eliminate all meat from my meals. This aided my anorexic behaviors in several ways. Now I could cleverly hide my disorder behind the new label of a "vegetarian." And with meat off limits in my new regimen, I could easily turn away from the bulk of most meals. If anyone made a comment about my meager intake, I could simply explain that I didn't eat meat and thus there were few options for me on the table.

My true hunger was for love. When did I convince myself that I did not deserve love? I believe this is a complication of the longevity of this illness. My doctor explains to me repeatedly that anorexia scares people away from intimacy. An anorexic offers an unpleasant and prickly embrace. Not only does any touch remind the other person that this individual is an unhealthy husk of bone, but touch invariably causes the anorexic to stiffen. I pulled into my shell whenever I sensed someone getting too close.

So over time I added "untouchable" to the list of adjectives I could use to describe myself. I understand this to be a word used in India for a person who can defile others through mere contact. This fit with my feelings about myself. I am sure there are parts of me that are spoiled and disgusting, and that contact with another person (most particularly anything that could be construed as "sexual" contact with a man) would bring ruin to the other person. I can prove this to myself by the fact that I have never had a man love me. I can still feel, however. I did not lose this sense. I only lost the appetite for it.

How many times over the years have I been admonished to come to my senses? I understood this to be criticism of my intellectual functioning. Now I know also that all five of my senses were dulled, but I am rediscovering the pleasures of them. Just as I can now enjoy eating some foods, I might learn to let touch excite rather than frighten me. It may be okay to want something. Just because I have never had it doesn't mean I can't ever have it.

Boldness

I am becoming bold. Slowly at first, taking tentative steps. The screamer inside me would have me stay back in a darkened corner, alone. But I move into the world anyway. For many years, I did not fully participate in my surroundings. I would sit in the back row at any meeting or class and never speak unless a question was directed specifically at me. If I didn't say anything, I couldn't say something stupid or wrong. Sometimes in a gathering I would even imagine myself to be quite invisible.

In the early years of my illness, when I was groping for a sense of control, I decided that there were two ways I could feel powerful: no one could make me eat, and no one could make me talk. Over the past few years, I have become more of a group participant. First, I developed the skill of listening; it's quite easy to find people who like to be listened to. And I practice asking questions. Inevitably I run into people who ask me questions in return. I am developing more ease with conversation. I have voluntarily joined groups and sometimes speak up about my ideas and opinions.

Boldness is a relative state. In a gray life, any glint of color looks vibrant. As the pounds dropped away from my body, I became a faded image. My speaking was often mumbled and my body language told everyone to leave me alone. I had the great fortune of living around people who valued life and were full of it, however. I feel thankful to these people for showing me by example that living can hold pleasure and wonder and be full of color.

It took me many, many years of meeting with my doctor before I could tell him about the negative thoughts in my head, and I am still working on letting him know each time they are ruling my behavior. This seems like more boldness on my part—to make it known to someone else that I am being ground into dirt. But when I am able to let him know that "I am being screamed at," I take much of the power away from that inner voice.

In the safety of therapy, I am testing my right to express opinions and experience disagreement. It has taken courage for me to let my doctor know (often a week after the fact) that I understood him to have said something I disagree with or that hurt my feelings in some way. The boldness here is twofold: first that I have enough conviction in my own belief to hold onto it, and second that disagreeing with him will not cause him to dislike me and kick me out of his office.

When I speak out now, I am often taken by surprise how forward I can be. Sometimes the words fly from my mouth before I have thought them through. Sometimes I even stumble over words. This can make others laugh. I can be funny! Mostly I just contribute to the normal daily give and take in speaking and listening. I am conversing again. I am living again.

Recovery

Anorexia brings only sadness and darkness and loss. So why is recovery from this illness so difficult? Why would anyone hang onto the destructive behaviors that characterize it? These are questions I ask but cannot answer—which, I believe, explains why this is an illness and not simply a passing phase or whim. There is nothing whimsical about anorexia. I am sorry that I have spent more than 20 years engaged in a battle with this tyrant. Yet fight I will, because anorexia's victory is death.

My steps are still hesitant. I am not fearless. There is much about recovery that I don't know yet, many risks still to be taken. But I now recognize that a full adult life is complex and unpredictable—very different from anorexic monotony. So recovery means breaking out into new territory. The old maps that I had and the ruts I used to follow no longer give me adequate guidance. I know there are difficult steps ahead of me, but I can look back and be encouraged by what I already gained.

I am far less tempted nowadays by the siren song of the cliff's edge, and much more interested in the rest of the journey that lies ahead of me. I move forward with curiosity and with a growing confidence that each step holds the promise of a wider view. I want to paint that view.

Night Falls Fast

By Kay Redfield Jamison, Ph.D.

Dr. Jamison is a professor of psychiatry at the Johns Hopkins University School of Medicine. She has received numerous awards and has studied extensively mood disorders, psychotherapy, and suicides. These excerpts are taken from her book Night Falls Fast, *which helps us understand suicide.*

Suicide has been a professional interest of mine for more than 20 years, and a very personal one for considerably longer. I have a hard-earned respect for suicide's ability to undermine, overwhelm, outwit, devastate, and destroy. As a clinician, researcher, and teacher, I have known or consulted on patients who hanged, shot, or asphyxiated themselves; jumped to their deaths from stairwells, buildings, or overpasses; died from poisons, fumes, prescription drugs, or slashed their wrists or cut their throats. Close friends, fellow students from graduate school, colleagues, and children of colleagues have done similar or the same. Most were young and suffered from mental illness; all left behind a wake of unimaginable pain and unresolvable guilt.

Like many who have manic-depressive illness, I have also known suicide in a private, awful way, and I trace the loss of a fundamental innocence to the day that I first considered suicide as the only solution possible to an unendurable level of mental pain. Until that time I had taken for granted, and loved more than I knew, a temperamental lightness of mood and a fabulous expectation of life. I knew death only in the most abstract of senses; I never imagined it would be something to arrange or seek.

I was seventeen when, in the midst of my first depression, I became knowledgeable about suicide in something other than an existential, adolescent way. For much of each day during several months of my senior year in high school, I thought about when, whether, where, and how to kill myself. I learned to present to others a face at variance with my mind, ferreted out the location of two or three nearby tall buildings with unprotected stairwells; discovered the fastest flows of morning traffic; and learned how to load my father's gun.

The rest of my life at the time—sports, classes, writing, friends, planning for college—fell fast into a black night. Everything seemed a ridiculous charade to endure; a hollow existence to fake one's way through as best one could. But, gradually, layer by layer, the depression lifted, and by the time my senior prom and graduation came around, I had been well for months. Suicide had withdrawn to the back squares of the board and become, once again, unthinkable.

Because the privacy of my nightmare had been of my own designing, no one close to me had any idea of the psychological company I had been keeping. The gap between private experience and its public expression was absolute; my persuasiveness to others was unimaginably frightening.

Over the years, my manic-depressive illness became much worse, and the reality of dying young from suicide became a dangerous undertow in my dealings with life. Then, when I was twenty-eight years old, after a damaging and psychotic mania, followed by a particularly prolonged and violent siege of depression, I took a massive overdose of lithium. I unambivalently wanted to die and nearly did. Death from suicide had become a possibility, if not a probability, in my life.

Under the circumstances—I was, during this, a young faculty member in a department of academic psychiatry—it was not a very long walk from personal experience to clinical and scientific investigation. I studied everything I could about my disease and read all I could find about the psychological and biological determinants of suicide. As a tiger tamer learns about the minds and moves of his cats, and a pilot about the dynamics of the wind and air, I learned about the illness I had and its possible end point. I learned as best I could, and as much as I could, about the moods of death.

Schizophrenia and the mood, anxiety, and personality disorders are at the heart of many suicides, but by no means all. Alcohol and drug abuse, either in their own right or, more commonly, in combination with depression and other mental illnesses, take a terrible toll as well. Substance abuse, like manic-depression and schizophrenia, usually begins early in life, often in adolescence or the early twenties, and once it has set in, has a stubbornly progressive course.

A few weeks after I nearly died from a suicide attempt, I went to the Episcopal church across the street from the UCLA campus. I was a parishioner there, however occasional, and in light of being able to walk in through the door instead of being carried in by six, I thought I would see what was left of my relationship with God. To make it easier, I purchased a ticket to a Bach recital that was being performed in the chapel. I went to the church early; my mind was still dull, and everything in it and in my heart was frayed and exhausted. But I knelt anyway, in spite of or because of this, and spoke into my hands the only prayer I really know or care very much about. The beginning was rote and easy: "God, be in my head, and in my understanding," I said to myself or God, "God, be in mine eyes, and in my looking." Somehow despite the thickening of my mind, I got through most of the rest of it. But then I blanked out entirely as I got to the end, struggling to get through what had started as an act of reconciliation with God. The words were nowhere to be found.

I imagined for a while that my forgetting was due to the remnants of the poisonous quantities of lithium I had taken, but suddenly the final lines came up into my consciousness: "God, be at mine end, and at my departing." I felt a convulsive sense of shame and sadness, a kind I had not known before, nor have I known it since. Where had God been? I could not answer the question then, nor can I answer it now. I do know, however, that I should have been dead but was not, and that I was fortunate enough to be given another chance at life, which many others were not.

I was naive to underestimate how disturbing it would be to write this book. I knew, of course, that it would mean interviewing people about the most painful and private moments of their lives, and I also knew that I would inevitably be drawn into my own private dealings with suicide over the years. Neither prospect was an attractive one, but I wanted to do something about the untolled epidemic of suicide and the only thing I knew to do was to write a book about it. I am by temperament an optimist, and I thought from the beginning that there was much to be written about suicide that was strangely heartening.

As a clinician, I believed there were treatments that could save lives; as one is surrounded by scientists whose explorations of the brain are elegant and profound, I believed our basic understanding of its biology was radically changing how we think about both mental illness and suicide; and as a teacher of young doctors and graduate students, I felt the future held out great promise for the intelligent and compassionate care of the suicidal mentally ill.

All of these things I still believe. Indeed, I believe them more strongly than I did when I first began doing background research for this book two years ago. The science is of the first water; it is fast paced, and it is laying down, pixel by pixel, gene by gene, the dendritic mosaic of the brain. Psychologists are deciphering the motivations for suicide and piecing

Finding Hope & Compassion

together the final straws—the circumstances of life—that so dangerously ignite the brain's vulnerabilities. And throughout the world, from Scandinavia to Australia, public health officials are mapping a clearly reasoned strategy to cut the death rate of suicide.

Still, the effort seems unhurried. Every seventeen minutes in America, someone commits suicide. Where is the public concern and outrage? I have become more impatient as a result of writing this book and am more acutely aware of the problems that stand in the way of denting the death count. I cannot rid my mind of the desolation, confusion, and guilt I have seen in the parents, children, friends, and colleagues of those who kill themselves. Nor can I shut out the images of the autopsy photographs of twelve-year-old children or the prom photographs of adolescents who, within a year's time, will put a pistol in their mouths or jump from the top floor of a university dormitory building. Looking at suicide—the sheer numbers, the pain leading up to it, and the suffering left behind—is harrowing. For every moment of exuberance in the science, or in the success of governments, there is a matching and terrible reality of the deaths themselves—the young deaths, the violent deaths, the unnecessary deaths.

Like many of my colleagues who study suicide, I have seen time and again the limitations of our science, been privileged to see how good some doctors are and appalled by the callousness and incompetence of others. Mostly, I have been impressed by how little value our society puts on saving the lives of those who are in such despair as to want to end them. It is a societal illusion that suicide is rare. It is not. Certainly the mental illnesses most closely tied to suicide are not rare. They are common conditions, and, unlike cancer and heart disease, they disproportionately affect and kill the young.

While writing this book, I kept on my desk a photograph and a fragment of a poem. The photograph is of a young, good-looking cadet at the Air Force Academy, standing next to a jet fighter. Writing about this young man's suicide was perhaps the most difficult part of writing this book. I started the essay on a clear winter day in the library at the University of St. Andrews in Scotland, where I teach for a few weeks each year. I was able to read his medical records only for brief periods before I had to get up, walk over to the window, and look out at the North Sea in a futile attempt to pull from it a meaning that would make more tolerable the awfulness of it all. I would then return to the medical notes that charted out the inexorable course of the illness that would kill him. The photograph at first haunted, then consoled me; I found great pleasure in knowing Drew Sopirak.

The fragment of the poem I kept on my desk was one that drew me to life. It was the last line from Douglas Dunn's "Disenchantments":

"Look to the living, love them, and hold on."

When Somebody Knows

By Rachel Naomi Remen, M.D.

The stories in Rachel Remen's book, My Grandfather's Blessings, *remind us that we all can comfort and bless others by smiling, listening, and showing that we care. Dr. Remen's professional knowledge and personal experience make her a very gifted counselor for people with chronic or terminal disease.*

I have had Crohn's disease for forty-seven years. In 1981, after feeling quite well for a long time, I began to have mysterious and frightening symptoms. Sometimes, in the midst of some ordinary activity, I would begin to shake uncontrollably, and within minutes my temperature would rise to 106. Other times I would grow flushed and experience the acute onset of such profound fatigue that, if I were out, I would barely be able to get home. My physicians ordered progressively more sophisticated tests without finding any answers. My numbers were normal, but I decidedly was not.

Over a period of several months, these symptoms grew more and more frequent and severe. I continued to visit my doctors regularly, more because I did not know what else to do than because I thought they could offer any explanation or help. Eventually I stopped telling them some of the more unusual things that I was experiencing. I felt they no longer wanted to hear.

As things became worse, I began to feel that something very dangerous was happening to me that no one could even name. The fear this caused is impossible to describe. It seemed to me that I was looking at the world through a plate glass window, caught up in a set of events that dominated my life, and that no one else experienced or understood. In desperation, I made an appointment to see yet another doctor, a surgeon who had sat with me on the advisory board of a research project.

Dr. Smith was the head of the department of surgery in a large HMO, a prepaid health plan whose protocol legislated the length of time that a doctor could spend with a patient during any single visit. We would have fifteen minutes together. Sitting and waiting in his tiny examining room, I regretted making this appointment. It would probably be a waste of time. What could this man possibly do to be of help in fifteen minutes when several other physicians had not been able to offer much, despite hours of their time?

There was a soft knock on the door and Dr. Smith entered. He greeted me and then spent a few minutes sitting quietly and reading over the lab results and X-ray studies I had brought with me. Then he leaned toward me and said, "Tell me why you have come…"

I looked into his face and saw a genuine concern. I began to tell him all the things I was experiencing, starting with the more commonplace and finally including such things as the strange taste that often awakened me from sleep, and the times when I suddenly lost all sense of direction and was unable to remember how to get home. My voice shook a little. He continued to listen.

Slowly I began to tell him other things, things I had not told anyone else—how the doctor who first diagnosed my illness had told me I would die before I was forty, that my father had unexpectedly died a few months previously because of a medication error and I had brought my mother, ill with severe heart disease, across the country to live with me. I shared my anxiety about being able to care adequately for her complex needs, the worry that my present health problems might cause me to let my own patients down, the loneliness I felt when friends went on without me because I could no longer keep up. Eventually I said it all and then I just cried.

It took no more than nine or ten minutes to tell my whole story. Dr. Smith said nothing to interrupt and just listened closely. When I had finished, he asked a few questions that showed me that he had heard and fully understood. Then he reached for my hand and told me that he realized how hard things were. He validated my concerns. Despite the strangeness of these happenings, this was not all in my head. "There is no question that there is something going on that we do not yet understand," he told me. He reminded me that my lab studies ruled out truly life-threatening possibilities. He assured me that, eventually, whatever this was would declare itself more clearly, and when it did, if there was a surgical solution, he would be there. He looked at me and smiled. "We will wait together," he told me.

Like the others, he had no diagnosis. What he offered was his caring and companionship, his willingness to face the unknown with me. In fourteen minutes he had lifted the loneliness that had separated me from others and from my own strength. In some way that I didn't understand then, this made all the difference. Someone else knew, someone else cared, and because of this, I found I had the courage to deal with whatever was going to happen.

Several months later, when the great abscess hidden deep in my abdomen finally appeared on an X-ray, it was he who did my surgery.

Jami Goldman

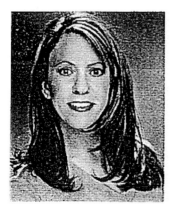

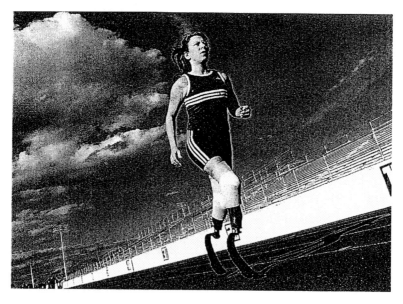

Photos by John Hall Photography

Up and Running

By Jami Goldman and Andrea Cagan

At age nineteen, Jami Goldman was trapped in the middle of a blizzard. After her rescue and in order to save her life, it became necessary to amputate both her frostbitten legs just below the knee. These excerpts from her inspiring book, Up and Running, *describe her recovery and eventual triumph over adversity. Happily married and a world-class athlete, she now feels that she is one of the luckiest women in the world.*

On December 23, 1987, I learned that a seemingly insignificant mistake can change the course of a person's life forever. I was driving home from a ski trip to spend the holidays with my family when I took a turn onto a seldom traveled road. That should have been no big deal. People get lost every day with repercussions no more serious than being late for an appointment. In my case, however, getting stuck on a back road that the state barricaded without first searching for travelers in distress wound up being costly beyond my wildest imagination.

After sliding into a snowbank on a deserted back road in Arizona in the middle of a blizzard, a friend and I were stranded in a red Chevy Mini-Blazer for eleven days without a telephone, heat, food, or water, besides small handfuls of snow we melted whenever the sun came out in bursts. When the intensity of the storm diminished, three days after we got stuck, we tried to escape by foot. Our plan was quickly thwarted when we fell into snow up to our knees. After pushing our way through the snow for a short distance, we were forced to retreat and take refuge back in the car. Little did I know that those were the last steps I would ever take on my own two feet. By the time we were found, we were half-delirious, freezing, frostbitten, thirsty beyond description, and wondering if we had been left for dead.

In another twenty-four to forty-eight hours, we would have died of dehydration, so as random and irreversible as my mistake was, when I open my eyes each morning and see my husband sleeping in bed beside me, I feel immensely grateful that I survived to tell my story. My friend, Lisa Barzano, a year younger than I, with whom I shared this life-altering experience, paid a tough price. After thirteen surgeries and the partial loss of several toes, she is in daily physical pain and is still healing from the emotional scars of those difficult days when we were lost, freezing and deprived. I bore a more dramatic physical burden. At age nineteen, after a painful and fruitless three-week therapeutic battle, I had both my legs amputated five inches below the knee. And yet, through the extraordinary love, caretaking, and steadfastness of my family, my friends, and my husband, Beau, I have healed emotionally, adjusted to life as a double below-the-knee amputee, and have become a decorated sprinter who sets world records and wins gold medals, and I am enthusiastic about my future.

Thirteen years after the fact, my original ordeal feels more like a dream than reality. Following seven weeks in the hospital, I returned home and deliberately placed the details of the accident into the background, as I had a daunting task ahead of me that required my full attention: learning to release what could have been, and to embrace life as a double amputee. I am grateful that human beings forget trauma faster than pleasure, but I have learned that we make peace with our past only when we achieve complete healing in the present. In this way, we can embrace the future with hope, joy, and strength of purpose.

Personal healing was a part of my motivation to write this book, but when I tried to recall my ordeal, the details had become vague in my memory, mainly because so many positive events had taken their place. And so I had to confer with the people who searched for me, found me, nursed me back to health, got me up on legs immediately, forced me to go to the gym, fitted me with prosthetics, taught me to walk again and finally to run like the wind, in order to spark my memory of the accident and the recovery period following.

No one will ever completely understand Lisa's and my eleven-day struggle for survival, or the massive adjustments that were required of me to reenter society as a whole woman. It's not that I consider my challenges to be more or less difficult than anyone else's. We all have our trials to bear in this life and mine have been considerable. But if the saying is true that living well is the best revenge, I have achieved my goals and then some. Each day when I get up in the morning, put on my legs and face a new day, I feel like one of the luckiest women in the world. My future children will, no doubt, agree.

Finding Hope & Compassion

Many years ago, during one of my first speaking engagements, a child stood up and asked me, "Do you want your legs back?" The truth is that, at the time, I would have given every penny I had or would ever attain, as well as all my material possessions, to feel my real legs beneath me. That was before I started running. Now I have a different point of view. I have found my purpose in life as an athletic amputee, an inspirational speaker, a role model for children and adults alike, and I wouldn't change a thing. When I'm sixty years old with my own grown kids and there is some groundbreaking surgery out there, I might decide that having legs would make life easier for me. For now, it's important for me to wake up and put on my prosthetics every day, because that defines for me who I am and where I am going.

The Real Bionic Woman

Running is a gift, plain and simple. The purest form of exhilaration I've ever known, it gives me a sense of freedom as I fly through the wind unencumbered, and a sense of achievement every time I cross a finish line. It's as if nothing can stop me as I push my body to the limit and I revel in the strength and power of my mind. I study other runners' styles, I listen to my coach for guidance, I watch videotapes to correct my mistakes, but when I run, I'm on my own, completely in control of my body and mind, and I like that.

Running also put me in touch with other disabled athletes and suddenly I had friends who faced the same kinds of challenges that I did. As soon as I started running, I got the sense that my life was in order and I came away from every competition with a little bit more of myself, unwilling to hide any aspect of who I was. The truth is that I love competing. I've always been a competitive person and I don't consider that a bad thing. It's part of my nature and brings out the best in me.

I practiced coming off the starting blocks, keeping my legs beneath me, determining the most efficient angle of my body, and I gained more confidence every day. When June arrived, I took my newfound confidence and my cheetah legs to compete in the U.S. Nationals in Springfield, Massachusetts.

The same sprinting legs that had started out as a source of great pain, between falls and giving me sores, had become my friends. I counted on them to propel me, support me, and allow me to move with tremendous speed and power. I learned to use their bionic capabilities to my advantage, as they afforded me the freedom to take my mind off speed and place it on technique. I marvel at them still, at how carbon fiber and metal has changed my life so dramatically and given me a new way to challenge myself and become a stronger and more capable human being.

Runners to Your Marks! Set!

I looked down at the ground in front of me, completely focused, waiting for the cracking sound that would start my legs moving and send me flying across the field. I had images of my training, my coach clapping her hands suddenly behind my head to help me get familiar with the gun. My cheetah legs were in position, I could hear my own breath, I could smell the track. Thirteen years ago, stranded on a lonely, deserted back road in Arizona in the middle of a blizzard, who could have predicted I would be here today, able to walk, able to run, able to compete fiercely in an athletic event? When you consider the way circumstances unfolded, the fact that I was alive at all was a miracle in itself....

Compassion

Nothing pleases me more than speaking to kids at their schools. Mostly I want to encourage kids to care about other people and to accept them for who they are—no matter how they look or what disabilities they might have. I led such a sheltered life when I was growing up. I wasn't exposed to people with different abilities. I don't remember anyone in my high school using a wheelchair, so I didn't have feelings for or against them. It just never came up. Today, the circumstances of my life have made me a more compassionate person and that has spilled over into the rest of my family. When my father sees a car parked in a disabled spot with no placard, he leaves a gentle reminder like a note on the windshield, reminding them that a disabled person might need that parking place. He never thought about it before, but it's amazing what a little awareness can do.

When I show the older kids my limbs, the oohs and aahs flow freely. They're so ready to accept new ideas, and they ask questions like, "Do your legs get rusty in the rain? Can you wiggle your toes? If you scratch an itch, does it really feel like you're scratching?" Then there is the all-important question that kids ask me so often: "Do you wish you had your legs back?"

I joke a little at first and say, "No way. Then I'd be short again." They laugh but the truth is that at this point in time, I would not want my legs back, and I tell them that. "I never would have chosen to lose them," I say, "but if I had my legs back right now, I wouldn't be sitting here, my life would have turned out completely differently, and I like it the way it is."

A child once asked me, "What's your job?" "Being here today is my job," I told her. "My life is my career." It's true. I wake up each day with appreciation and I get ready to accept my life exactly as it is and to take care of business. Whether that means going to the gym, giving a speech, or seeing the prosthetist or the doctor, my goal is to put a smile on my face and to be present for my life, just like anybody else. That's what I want to impress on the kids, that we don't always get to choose the circumstances of our lives but we do get to choose our attitudes. If I can be a positive role model for kids and teach them to have compassion for other people, especially for those less fortunate than they, I will have put in a good day's work.

People say to me, "I never could have survived what you did. I would have fallen apart."

I once heard an adage that goes something like: Do not judge another man until you have walked a mile in his shoes. I haven't walked a mile in your shoes and you definitely haven't walked in mine. No matter what you might imagine, there's no way to know how you would handle what happened to me. If anyone ever told me I would have to give up my perfect little legs, the only small things about me besides my height, I never would have thought I could go on. But I have gone on; we all do, each in our own way, and I think people have the wrong impression of me. There are times I wake up in the morning and I bitch and complain—just ask Beau. I say things like, "I don't want to put on my legs; I don't want to go to the track today." And when I get to the track, I'm annoyed about having to go through the long process of changing my legs, making sure they're right when I start running, and then going through tearing a sleeve or falling down and getting a bruise. Sometimes it puts me in a bad mood. I'm only human; I have my off days, and I can be plenty crabby. But I move beyond it and try to remember that I'm alive. It usually brings me back.

I don't know what your individual trials are—they may be a lot worse than mine—and I can't tell you how to handle a crisis. That comes in the moment, and I hope you never have to find out. The one thing we all have in common is our capacity to open our hearts. So if you want to have compassion for others and for yourself, I can tell you who I am, what I've done for myself, and how I access my energy and strength. I can also let you know what your support does for me. If any of that helps, I'm happy to offer it.

On April 28, 2001, I married Beau Marseilles, the love of my life, under the setting sun in Scottsdale, Arizona. Little Savannah, my flower girl, had just finished strewing the white carpet with rose petals so slowly and meticulously, Brittney, her mom and my maid of honor, had to urge her daughter to keep walking forward amid peals of laughter from family and friends. If she had continued at her snail's pace, loath to leave the limelight, we might have been there all night. I wouldn't have minded; I'd waited my whole life to be right where I was, so what difference would a few more hours make.

I have no idea what's coming next in my own life, which is what makes it so compelling. But in the spirit of Mrs. Lindbergh, I can only say that whatever it is, nobody has to worry about me. I'm ready, I'm waiting, and I'm up and running.

Dan and Judy Miller

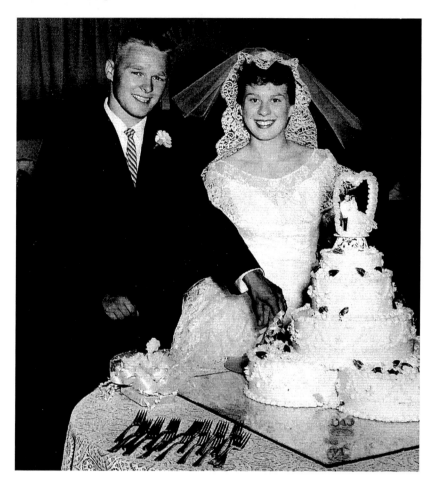

Photo by Ron Gies

From Judy: On August 15, 1959, I married that man. To this day he continually surprises me with his approach to the world and people in it. He brings joy and happiness to our lives and a richness that I never could have imagined. He is still cute and has a twinkle in his eyes. He has never been a little man. He is a giant!

Living, Laughing, and Loving Life

By Dan Miller

Dan Miller had crippling polio at age 18 but, supported by family and friends, has achieved remarkable goals, including successful careers as a teacher and an elementary school principal. His three children and wife Judy love Dan's sense of humor and their challenging, adventurous life together.

Dan, who has weakness in one arm and 80 percent paralysis of both legs, learned how to swim, play golf, shoot basketball hoops, ride a motorcycle, and, believe it or not, fly a plane. He also played and sang in a band and taught guitar lessons.

Dan began full-time speaking in 1990 and has shared his message of hope with many people. His book Living, Laughing and Loving Life *reminds us that we should enjoy life and not lose sight of our dreams in spite of the difficulties that face us.*

Five weeks after high school graduation, I contracted polio. For the next 15 months I was enrolled in two unexpected classes of life. I called them Physical Therapy 101 and Rehab 102. The legs that sprang for rebounds were now 80 percent paralyzed. The right arm that propelled jump shots was virtually useless. My left arm, which now gripped an elbow-high Canadian crutch, had about half of its original muscle.

I no longer had an athlete's body as I began that slippery trip to the college field house that cold December day. My registration packet was labeled "P.E. exempt." I was so unsteady that I fell a half-dozen times trying to find the physical education professor assigned as my advisor.

I'm not sure what Dr. Richard Hagelin first thought as I wobbled into his office and plopped into a chair. I can't run or jump, I told him, as I dropped my crutch. I can't do push-ups or pull-ups. I can't climb a rope or jump rope, but I want to major in physical education and become a P.E. teacher.

I now wonder if he knew how much the rest of my life would hinge on his response. I knew he could say, "I'm sorry, Danny, you're in the wrong department." I couldn't lift either arm above my head. I couldn't throw a football or shoot a basket. I had no athletic skills and he knew it. But he didn't hesitate a moment. He just smiled and said, "Well, let's see what you can do."

One day I decided to walk to the locker room and gym to soak up some good athletic smells. Between the locker room and gym was a ramp. As I went up, I lost my balance and fell. I couldn't get up, and there was no one around to help me. A high school teacher soon came by, and we had a nice little chat. I think she was too embarrassed to ask if I needed help. I was too embarrassed to ask for assistance. I've noticed some people do not know how to handle situations like this so they avoid them if they can.

After she left, I was wondering how I would get up when a little sixth grader came along and asked, "Hey, you need help?" A sixth grader! Yup, he helped me up and I was on my way.

People stared, but I had learned to accept my body and ignore their stares. When others made fun of me or my physical limitations, I decided they were the ones who were limited, not me. I realized my friends and family loved me because of who I was and how I treated them, not on the basis of what I looked like. I accepted myself the way I was.

I guess I represent thousands who have dealt with handicaps. I know the frustrations of being a one-armed, weak-legged person. Sometimes even putting on a belt can be aggravating. Just try reaching around your waist with one arm and putting that belt through the loops! A lot of fix-it or mechanical jobs are too much for me. I know how, but they are two-handed tasks. I can't hold a nail in one hand and pound with a hammer with the other. It's no fun taking an hour on a job that should take ten minutes because you have to hold something with your teeth or figure out another way to do it with one hand.

Although there are many things I cannot do, or which are very difficult to do, I am thankful for what I have. My focus has not been on what I can't do but on what I can do.

I didn't always think of my handicap as a "gift," but now I see how it has changed my life for the better. My life has been filled with wonderful, caring people and challenging adventures that I would have missed as a "normal" person. I have lived an exciting, abundant life here on earth. And because my relationship with God will last forever, I have an eternity of wonderful Mondays to look forward to.

Finding Hope & Compassion

Bill and Margaret Flannery

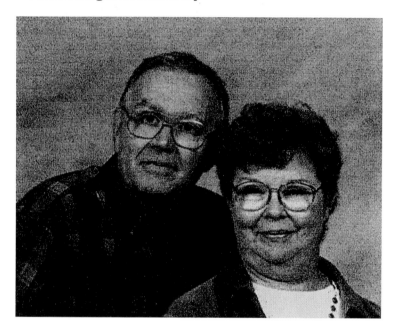

Author's photo

Finding Hope & Compassion

Courage Is in the Eye of the Beholder

By Margaret E. Flannery
Introductory Commentary by Burton Sack, M.D.

I have had the pleasure of caring for Margaret Flannery for 21 of the 23 years she has suffered with rheumatoid arthritis. Despite my best efforts and the latest new therapies that became available, I was only able to accomplish temporary remissions. Remissions slow or stop the progressive destruction of the "malignant" inflammation. Margaret unfortunately is one of a small percentage of rheumatoids who have a relentless downhill course, despite best efforts.

She was on drugs that were supposed to slow or stop the damage. When a joint would flare, I would inject it with cortisone, relieving the pain and inflammation until another joint flared. But I repeatedly had to refer her to surgery because the damage had gone too far. She had both shoulders and one hip replaced. Damaged joints in her feet were removed. Her thumb joints were fused to allow a good pincer grip. Ruptured tendons in her hands were repaired. She is now facing a neck operation because loosening has put her spinal cord in jeopardy. The neck problem was found when she was being evaluated pre-op for corrective elbow surgery.

It is possible that Margaret would have fared even worse had it not been for her medications, but I don't know that. But there is some comfort in knowing that at least I was there to help her when she was in pain, to educate her, and to make clinical judgments when surgery was needed.

Margaret is a very courageous and wonderful person. She is never preoccupied or unduly depressed by her condition. I have been frustrated that the available technologies I offered her failed, but I learned from Margaret that medicine is more than offering technologies. She made me realize that medicine is an art of "being there to comfort." Hopefully the new technologies being developed based on increased knowledge of this disease will help others with this condition. I have always liked Margaret and consider her a close friend. I wish I could have helped her more.

I consider myself a very lucky person. I had a very happy, healthy childhood, filled with experiences of which many children today only dream. I was always secure in the knowledge of my parents' love for me. I was blessed with blue eyes, blond hair, a pretty face and reasonable intelligence—but not much common sense. Thank Heaven I had good parents! With the exception of a brief six-week battle with poliomyelitis in 1955 at the age of 12, which I took in stride, every chapter in my life was right out of a storybook—as "normal" as apple pie. Then something went wrong.

In 1980 when I was 37, and couldn't stand any longer the mysterious pain in my feet, knees and wrists, I finally gave in and sought the help of a physician. I had always been a physically active person, enjoying hiking, biking, skating, swimming, tennis, and the like. I couldn't understand what was happening to me. When my doctor told me I had rheumatoid arthritis, I was ignorant of the disease or the impact that diagnosis would have on me. I remember writing to my brother with the bad news, saying that with medical help I'd be back on the tennis court in no time. Little did I know. I haven't held a racquet since.

It took me some time to accept my "fate" and decide to somehow take charge of the situation. My rheumatologist, Burton Sack, a compassionate and conservative doctor, guided me through every step of combating this disease, and instilled in me a confidence that there is always hope. He always considers my complaints as legitimate and recommends a remedy. I, therefore, avoid casual complaining, sometimes to the point of not saying enough, since I consider my lesser symptoms as par for the course. With a thorough knowledge of rheumatology as well as general medicine, Dr. Sack has kept himself up to date with the latest advances. We tried many medications over the next 20 years, each in its order of potency and often in combination. They would work for a while then lose their efficacy or cause unpleasant side effects. The latest, Enbrel, seems to be working, but much painful damage has already been done.

Joints would continue to become severely and painfully damaged. Numerous fluid aspirations of each knee, repair of ruptured tendons in the right hand, and finally further surgical intervention was the only answer to make my life more bearable. First both shoulders were replaced, then the right hip, and much later the left knee. My right elbow, both feet, and both hands also required further surgery.

The hip replacement proved to be pain free but unstable, it having dislocated about 13 times to date. A broken left humerus required a total left shoulder revision. And now I've been told I need to have the top two vertebrae in my neck fused to my skull, a risky procedure.

Somehow, through it all, I have never given up hope, maintaining a sense of humor. I think I simply go from day to day, optimistic that soon things will get easier, or at least stop getting worse. I don't really know the

Finding Hope & Compassion

source of my courage or determination to cope with the unrelenting de- structive nature of this disease. Looking back, I have to say my ability must have been in me all along, God given, and it gradually emerged through the loving patience of a wonderful husband, a bright son who still makes me laugh (especially at myself), and terrific parents. My mother's quiet strength and deep, abiding faith would later prove to be inspirational to me when I needed something more to lean on for strength and comfort. She planted the seed of faith in God's love and grace in me when I was a child, and by her example has awakened in me a realization that a sustaining faith is es- sential for my overall well-being.

My ability to cope must be a sort of defense mechanism, a survival technique that took hold and surprised even me without any conscious ef- fort on my part. I have, however, kept myself well informed, asking ques- tions of doctors, seeking information from the Arthritis Foundation, joining support groups, arthritis aquatics and exercise programs, and taking an ac- tive role in managing my health.

It took me a while to accept help and support from those outside my immediate family—friends, clergy, etc. So many wonderful supportive people have told me what spirit I have, what an amazingly cheerful attitude I have through all this adversity. To me this is simply "my life." I want to live it to the best of my ability, and at the same time not alienate those around me with constant complaining and self-pity. I don't mourn the things I have lost, but am rejuvenated by the happy memories and rejoice in what I do have.

I am thankful for the joy many things give me—a warm evening breeze as I sit on my front porch listening to the spring peepers, sunsets, ocean surf on a sandy shore, hearing my husband laugh, looking into the beautiful clear blue eyes of my four-year-old granddaughter, delighting in the impish grin of my little 16-month-old grandson, good music, being an American—to name a few.

This is not to say that I have surrendered to this disease or any other. I still have my moments when I have to have a really good cathartic cry—scream, rant and rave out of sheer frustration for my diminishing abil- ity to do even the simplest tasks around the house, or take a walk in the woods or on the beach with my husband. Every day is a struggle of one kind or another. Some days are better than others. I allow myself the luxury of rest when I need it to regroup my resources of strength, and then I move on.

It has never occurred to me to give up but to accept each new challenge, stubbornly optimistic, and to make the most of the situation. As a favorite activity becomes difficult or impossible to do, I either find another way to do it, or find something new that gives me pleasure and a sense of accomplishment. Most notable is my learning how to use a computer. I took courses to learn the basics, and with my son's knowledgeable assistance, acquired the best hardware and software for my purposes. He has always pushed me to learn how to use it on my own, but helps troubleshoot any problems I encounter. He keeps me challenged though. Once I get accustomed to a new hardware or software upgrade, he wants to upgrade me again. I guess I must be getting old—I understand old people don't like change.

I once enjoyed creating things out of wood, having built my young son a sandbox and an easel. I even tried my hand at oil and watercolor painting. Since being a carpenter or holding a brush or standing at an easel are now unachievable, I enjoy creating on the computer as newsletter editor for two organizations. It has given me a real sense of accomplishment, for I taught myself how to design layouts and write articles. I also often design my own greeting cards on the computer, incorporating scanned photos I want to share. The computer has also helped me keep up my correspondence with distant family and friends through e-mail, since handwriting a letter has become tedious and the writing barely legible.

My most recent vocation was secretary and bookkeeper, first for my church parish and then for a local businessman in his cottage industry. When I had to stop working, I felt nonproductive and felt a need to do something useful or helpful. To fill that need I accepted several positions as secretary, treasurer, or publicity chairman for local organizations to which I belong. I even enjoyed the privilege of being regent (president) of my DAR chapter for six years, a position I never would have aspired to in my younger days.

I used to enjoy gardening—getting my hands dirty, watching things grow. I now enjoy nurturing houseplants, watching them grow. When they turn brown, I simply start over. I have taken up contract bridge again, something I learned in college, even though holding 13 cards in my hand and dealing are difficult, and shuffling is impossible. My bridge friends shuffle for me and wait patiently as I sort my "hand," even when my partner and I are winning.

Cabinet shelves and the deep, dark recesses of my refrigerator (where unidentifiable leftovers grow green and fuzzy) are totally out of my reach. Tight screw caps, milk cartons, cellophane packages, cereal boxes are all a real challenge for me to open. I employ a number of gadgets to assist me—scissors, knives, jar opener, pop-top lifter, my teeth, etc.—but it is frustrating nonetheless. Now my meal preparation consists of the minimum necessary for nourishment, and we eat out for enjoyment.

We have always enjoyed traveling, and in spite of difficulty walking and ascending stairs, we continue to travel, arranging our trips around wheelchair accessibility. The kindness of strangers and the helpfulness of the travel industry have made all of our trips wonderful experiences.

Family and friends are so willing to help in any way they can, beyond my wildest expectations. I often wonder that if the tables were turned, would I be such a kind and generous person to help those in need? I certainly hope so. I can say for certain that the desire to do so is far stronger in me now than it ever was before, though it bothers me that I most likely will never be able to reciprocate in kind. I have learned to be less judgmental of others, putting aside preconceived notions, something my husband has always been able to do. I have become far less self-centered and self-conscious and more sympathetic and outgoing, but there is still room for improvement.

In conclusion, I feel one's courage is personal and relative to the sacrifices and burdens one must bear. Each one of us has courage all our own. One person's burden overcome may be beyond the comprehension of another, but the latter is no less courageous. To paraphrase two familiar adages that help me put my life in perspective: first, the Lord seldom gives us a burden beyond our capacity to bear it, and second, do not grieve because you have no shoes; think of the man who has no feet.

Art Berg

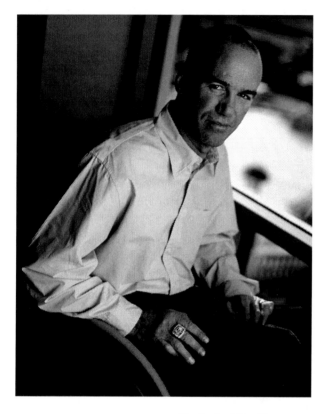

Photo by Tim Mantoani

The race was grueling; 325 miles in 7 days through the Utah hills. "Tough but doable," Art says. Art Berg is a quadriplegic who is unable to use his legs. Now he is a competitive wheelchair racer.

To the Top: The Difficult Takes Time; the Impossible Takes a Little Longer

By Art Berg

Art Berg broke his neck in a car accident, becoming a quadriplegic who would never be able to use his legs again. Now he is a competitive wheelchair racer and an inspirational speaker. Art is married and has two children. This excerpt was published in the April 2002 issue of Guideposts.

Quickly I made one last check of my equipment at the starting line: half-finger racing gloves Velcroed on firmly, helmet secure, wrist taped tight. I leaned over into my racing tuck and got ready to go. From the corner of my eye, I saw the starter raise his pistol, a dark metallic outline against the vivid blue Utah sky. Stealing a glance toward the sidelines, 1 spotted my family and friends, ready to explode into cheers at the sound of the gun. Later, along the grueling 325 miles and the seven days it was supposed to take to complete this wheelchair race from Salt Lake City to St. George, they would act as my support crew. No quadriplegic with my level of paralysis had ever attempted such a marathon, let alone finished. Now, though, I just needed a last peek at my family—including my wife Dallas, who'd been at my side since that terrible day late in 1983.

We were still engaged back then, and I was riding in a friend's car from California to Utah to be with her for the Christmas holidays. I was 21, had my own tennis court construction company and was in top physical shape. Golf, bowl, ski—you name it. I liked to compete and I liked to succeed. I was young, confident, and ambitious. I believed that God had great plans for my future.

That was before the car flipped over on a lonely stretch of highway in the Nevada desert. I came to in the intensive care unit of a hospital following four hours of emergency surgery. A doctor standing at my bedside leaned over and said, as gently as he could, "Art, you have broken your neck in a car accident. You are a quadriplegic."

I stared unblinking at the ceiling. I was supposed to get married in five weeks. *Lord, this can't be happening to me.*

The doctor laid out the facts: I would never regain use of my legs; I'd lost most of the use of my arms and shoulders; I would require help dressing, eating, going to the bathroom, and getting around; I would be on medication for as long as I lived, which would be considerably less than normal. The bottom line: I would spend my life in a wheelchair.

"I'm sorry, Art. You are going to have to think new thoughts, dream new dreams."

What dreams could I possibly have left except nightmares?

My mother soon arrived at my bedside from California. The hopelessness in my eyes must have been plain to her. She took one of my limp hands firmly in hers and squeezed. "I know things look bleak and impossible right now," she said. "But I promise we'll all help you, Art. Things will get better." Then she added something I'd never heard before, something I have never forgotten. "While the difficult takes time, the impossible just takes a little longer."

Her words only made me feel a little better, but it was something. It was a start, a glimmer of hope that would have to grow if I were to survive.

Soon my fiancée Dallas arrived. We'd been together since we were young teens when our families met on a ski vacation in Utah. I always knew we'd spend the rest of our lives together. Now, though...

"Art," she whispered, laying her check gently on my chest. "We'll get through this. Together. That's why God led us to each other."

I needed all of my family's prayers and support to face the doubt and despair that inevitably set in when your life is suddenly torn down. I dwelled obsessively on what I'd lost—my career, my future, my freedom. I was a prisoner of a wheelchair, a hulking chrome monstrosity weighing some 65 pounds. My hands couldn't grip, so I had to push the wheels with the heels of my palms. It was agonizing. I barely made progress. "Listen, Art," my physical therapist advised, "you'd be much better off in an electric wheelchair."

That's when it happened, my old stubborn competitive streak kicked in. No! I would not give in. I would not surrender my last vestige of physical autonomy. I would leave that hospital under my own power, even if I were in a chair. *I know you will help me, Lord.*

One day my doctors and therapists laid out an eighth-of-a-mile course on the first floor. If I could complete it in less than 30 minutes, I could avoid what I'd grimly termed "the electric chair."

My fiancée walked by my side down the first long corridor. "You're doing fantastic, honey," she marveled. Maybe I pushed too hard at the beginning. Halfway through, my arms and shoulders started to ache. They felt as weak as when I woke up in intensive care, before months of grueling physical therapy. Sweat ran down my temples. You used to run three miles a day! If I couldn't do this, what was left for me? I would lose everything. Just as my arms cramped up, I crossed the finish line to the cheers of the staff, 28 minutes flat. I shouted as if I had just captured Olympic gold. Dallas kissed me. "I knew you could do it!"

I think that eighth of a mile was the most important distance I have ever traveled, except perhaps up the church aisle with her a year later. I set out to disprove the assumptions made about how many major life functions a person with my level of injury could regain. I went into business with my brother-in-law and did very well, well enough to eventually sell the business and become a motivational speaker, appearing at youth conferences and summer camps. Dallas and I had kids. My life exceeded what doctors had predicted for me. Indeed I had had new thoughts and dreamed new dreams. Yet there was still some old stuff kicking around, something that had simmered since I beat the clock on the eighth-of-a-mile course in the hospital. I yearned to compete physically again.

One day at a family picnic, everyone was playing croquet. I couldn't stand it. "I want in," I finally demanded. By then people knew better than to stop me. A friend taped a mallet to my arm, then wheeled me around the yard while I swung away. Mostly I gouged divots in my sister's lawn, but I had a blast.

I'd heard about wheelchair racing. Among its practitioners, it was a very serious sport. Though most wheelchair racers are paraplegics—they have full use of their arms—I became convinced I could compete as a quadriplegic who'd regained some upper body function. "They told me to dream new dreams," I said to my mother. "Well?"

I started training, pushing myself every day, building up my arm strength, until I was ready for my first race, a five-miler. I rolled across the finish line in two and one-half hours—dead last by at least an hour. I trained harder and entered more races, working on stamina. Two years later I finished a 10K race—6.2 miles—in under an hour. The next year I did a marathon—26.2 miles—in less than three hours. I was ready for the ultramarathon from Salt Lake to St. George, as ready as I'd ever be.

I took one last look at my family. A few minutes before I had gotten into position at the starting line, we'd formed a prayer circle. Now I said a prayer of my own, then concentrated my gaze down the center of the road. I tried to block out my doubts. Mom's words came back to me—the impossible just takes a little longer. This would take seven days up and down some of Utah's steepest mountains. The starting gun sounded. I was off.

Nothing I had ever attempted compared to the sheer physical effort of this race. I pushed myself mercilessly. I screamed, I cried, I prayed. At night I would rest, but at dawn I was back out on the course. By the third day, despite my sleek black racing suit and the electric pink tank top, I was not looking too good. My arms and shoulders were going numb. My doctor, who was trailing me along with my sister Beverly, finally said, "Call it quits, Art. Why risk permanent damage?"

I chuckled and looked down at my legs, "Permanent damage?" I asked.

"All right," he said. "Just promise me you'll stop if it gets too bad. You don't have anything to prove."

Day four brought headwinds so stiff I had to push even going downhill. *I know I can do this. I know you will help me, Lord.* Yet the doubts came on. Am I crazy? Is it too much? Day five arrived with brutal heat—105 degrees. My family took turns dousing me with cold water. Soon my muscles were beyond fatigue. I no longer even had the strength to talk. I leaned forward, closed my eyes and pushed. One hour. Two. Three.

Somewhere in those long hot hours I heard footsteps crunching in the gravel next to me. I assumed it was Beverly. I stayed silent and kept my gaze focused ahead, not daring to let up. Each footfall gave me a spurt of energy, a sense of calm and renewed strength, a feeling of complete peace in the midst of complete physical exhaustion. All at once I understood. I'd finally broken through that wall which so many other marathoners talk about. I was on the other side and now the race seemed doable. Tough, but definitely doable.

Finally I raised my head to say thanks. No one was there. I glanced over my shoulder. Beverly was pedaling her bike, lagging at least 30 yards back. I looked all around and realized the footsteps in the gravel had stopped as suddenly as they had started.

Finding Hope & Compassion

I had one daunting challenge ahead: a 9,000-foot climb before the downhill homestretch. On day seven it took me a full 13 hours to make it up, literally foot by foot. I kept thinking about that eighth of a mile back at the hospital, with my family and friends urging me on. At one point I nearly careened into a gully backward. When I reached the top, I finally allowed myself to rest for a moment, staring out at the vast craggy landscape spread before me, stretching for what seemed like eternity. Sitting back in my racing chair, I felt as if I was 21 years old again. Yes, God had great plans for my future.

I tightened my helmet and started the long fast descent into St. George. The breeze made me feel weightless, like I was flying, and I gave thanks.

Lisa I. Iezzoni, M.D., M.Sc.

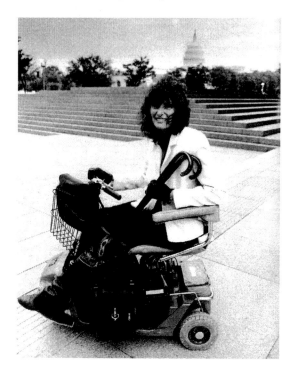

Photo by Mark L. Rosenberg, M.D., M.P.P.

What Should I Say? Communication around Disability

On Being a Patient

By Lisa I. Iezzoni, M.D., M.Sc.

Dr. Iezzoni is a professor of medicine at Harvard Medical School in the Division of General Medicine and Primary Care, Beth Israel Deaconess Medical Center, East Campus, Boston, Massachusetts. She has multiple sclerosis, uses a wheelchair, and enjoys being as independent as possible, serving on national committees, using her computer, and giving inspirational speeches. She is uniquely qualified to share her insights on disability and how to improve communication with those who are disabled. The following essay appeared in the Annals of Internal Medicine 1998; 129:661-665, *and was adapted from an article in the October 1998 issue of the* Harvard Medical Alumni Bulletin.

Every so often, we all experience moments that crystallize an essential truth about our lives. Last spring, I had one in the cramped interstices of a federal office building in Washington, D.C. Before a meeting, I hurried to a back office to use the telephone, but a man was already there. We recognized each other instantly.

"It's been 20 years," I said. "You taught that great course on patients' experiences of illness. It helped me decide to go to medical school."

"I remember you well." He paused, eyeing me with momentarily unguarded sadness. "I heard about your troubles."

My mind raced. What troubles? Instantaneously a student again, I wondered what this professor could mean. Academic troubles? That would be too awful! Then I understood. "Oh, you mean my multiple sclerosis (MS)? I don't think of that as trouble. I'm doing fine!"

We spoke telegraphically, catching up, until my meeting began. Later, I rolled out onto the mall below the Capitol. The day was glorious, but I could think only of the encounter with my former professor. My reaction puzzled me. Why had I not immediately understood what he meant by "your troubles"? I felt that he was saddened to see me in a wheelchair; when he knew me 20 years ago, I ran everywhere. I also sensed that he wanted to hide his sorrow. This worried me; I didn't want to distress him. Why was I compelled to reassure him I was fine? His look also conveyed admiration, something that makes me uncomfortable. Given the alternative, what could I do but go on? And, yes, what I told him was true. My MS does not feel like "trouble"—just the landscape I live in. How had I arrived at this point?

Subtexts

Although this encounter held many layers of meaning for me, one aspect is shared by all persons with visible disabilities: the implicit embargo on spoken words and the volumes of unspoken thoughts permeating our relationships with others, even our passing greetings. Communicating around disability is hard on both sides. People often don't know what to say or where to look. Silence frequently subsumes a complex tangle of fears, discomforts, and uncertainties. Other times, similarly complicated feelings prompt spoken words of many stripes: generous, tentative, hurtful, intrusive. As Sally Ann Jones, a woman with MS, said to me, "Some people see you're in a wheelchair and immediately they raise their voice as if you are deaf. I mean, you're some kind of handicapped. They're not quite sure what to do. People aren't comfortable with handicapped people."

For those of us with disabilities, silence is often the default position. We ourselves are uncomfortable talking about our disability, concerned about breaching that invisible barrier circumscribing socially acceptable discourse. We think, generally erroneously, that silence protects our previous privacy.

But silence carries consequences. As Mrs. Jones said, "In some ways, it's your obligation to kind of educate them and make them more comfortable." Silence reinforces the stigmatization of disability, the sense of shame and guilt, and the idea that disability is something to hide. Nonetheless, opening communication around disability is difficult. What should I say? What should you say to me? One place to start is with examples of communication gone awry—what not to say or do. I have innumerable examples taken from my experiences and from stories told to me.

Failed Communication

Becoming Invisible

Persons in wheelchairs live below the eye level of most standing adults. Nonetheless, something other than this physical fact must make us sometimes invisible. Positioned strategically in full view of others, we often remain unnoticed. One example of this phenomenon involved a physician colleague, Megan Martin. After Megan had a complex metatarsal fracture, her orthopedist insisted that she stay off her foot for six weeks. I encountered Megan on her return to work and she was frantic. Her clinical and administrative offices were far apart; on crutches, the trip had taken 45 minutes and she was exhausted. How could she manage the multiple trips per day that were required? The solution seemed obvious. "Why don't you rent a scooter like mine," I suggested.

As I expected—and fully understood—Megan's initial response was unenthusiastic. "People will think I am a wimp," she worried. I did not argue; certainly they would. "I'll think I'm a wimp." That was undoubtedly true, too. In two days, she had rented a scooter. Later, Megan acknowledged that she couldn't have managed without the scooter, but she had remained uncomfortable and rarely left the building in it.

"[It's as if] you're not there. The few times I did take it out, it was almost impossible to get through a crosswalk before the light changed. People are crossing in front of you. I'd be sitting right at the curb, waiting to go, and somebody would walk right in front of me and then just stand there and chat for a while. Well, *they* can run when the light changes. I thought, this is crazy. People don't want to see you; they're not going to see you… "

One day after the six weeks had ended, Megan was standing outside my office, balanced on crutches. Nick, another physician and a nice man, approached her. "Megan, did you do something to your foot," he asked. Nick had been around when Megan had been using the scooter. How could he not have noticed? Megan told me afterward that many people reacted the same way. They did not inquire about her injury while she used the scooter, but when she resumed the use of crutches, they asked whether she had hurt herself.

"It was amazing. It wasn't apparent what was going on until the day I was upright. And then it just hit me. Everybody knows *now*. Finally, they're noticing I've got a broken foot. It went from as if I weren't there one day, and all of a sudden I'd come back after being absent for a month. The whole time it was really uncomfortable for people."

Seen but Not Heard

Although seen, sometimes we are not heard. For example, returning to Boston after a business trip, a colleague pushed my airport-issue wheelchair to the gate. The agent processed our tickets and addressed my colleague.

"Here's a sticker to put on her coat," the agent said, gesturing toward me with a round, red-and-white-striped sticker.

"Why?" I asked.

"It will alert the flight attendants that she needs help," the agent replied to my colleague.

"Thanks. If need help, I'll ask for it."

"But the sticker indicates she needs assistance." My bemused colleague remained silent.

"When I need help, I'll ask for it."

"So she won't wear the sticker?"

"No, I won't."

"Why won't she?"

"Because I can ask for help."

"Why won't she wear it?"

This was going nowhere. I looked up at my colleague, imploring her to stop this silliness. "Because it's demeaning," she said and rolled me away.

Not Asking

Admittedly, many people with disabilities hesitate to ask for help. We are often proudly self-sufficient, and requesting assistance is hard. Sometimes we are stopped by implicitly being on the lower rung of that inevitable hierarchy of human relationships. In these instances, the right thing would be for the other person to ask us what we need, as suggested by these two examples:

A colleague, Andrea Banks, told me about her patient, a young man with progressive debility from cerebral palsy. He uses a wheelchair and is brought to appointments by his aunt. Andrea said that the first few times she examined him, she had him sit in his wheelchair rather than get up on the examining table. She thought that would be easier for him, but she never asked him if that was what he wanted. One day, the nurse told Andrea that the patient's aunt had complained, "Dr. Banks never even asked my nephew to walk to see how he does." The patient and his aunt were concerned that his walking had grown worse, and they wondered how Andrea could evaluate this when she had never seen him walk.

During a third-year clerkship in medical school, my MS flared up. I could no longer use the stairs when rounds with the attending physician traveled among beds scattered across several floors. As the team entered the stairwell, I went to the elevators, hoping to arrive at the next floor in time to see the team down the hallway en route to the next room. I was still in my "tough-it-out, don't-talk-about-it" mode, but it nonetheless hurt that neither the attending nor the residents seemed to notice my visible difficulty in walking and left me behind. I was also timid. At that point, my attendings seemed to hold my destiny in their hands. I did not speak up until the attending paused during the closing of a fairly brutal exit interview at the end of his month.

"Didn't you notice I was having trouble walking?" I ventured.

"I did," he responded. "But because I understood you wanted to be treated just like other students, I didn't ask."

Saying Too Much

Persons with physical disabilities are frequently grabbed or touched by persons unknown and unasked. In general, this seems to be motivated by genuine efforts to help. Sometimes it preserves our physical safety, as it did when I was lifted off a busy Washington, D.C., street by several strangers after my wheelchair tipped over in a pothole. Nonetheless, unrequested physical contact can be unnerving and physically uncomfortable. Similarly, conversation can cross acceptable boundaries even if others are trying to be kind.

For example, late one evening during a third-year clerkship, I was completing my write-up at the deserted nurses' station. The new resident approached me with instructions, making it obvious that he was unaware of my situation; because of the risks posed by extreme fatigue, my neurologists refused to allow me to take call. I had asked the clerkship director to communicate this to my supervisors because I was shy and embarrassed.

When I informed the resident of my situation, he instantly responded with a barrage of questions. What neurologic tracts were involved? Was I incontinent of urine? Of stool? My legs were tremulous and, yes, I was concerned about driving home. I answered dispassionately, as if making a clinical presentation. Apparently satisfied as to the nature of my impairment, the resident led me, virtually by the hand, out the front door of the hospital and to the taxi stand. He placed me in a cab, telling the driver to take me home and to return the next morning at 6:00 a.m. to bring me back. The resident paid the driver a generous sum. Despite this somewhat surreal interchange, the resident's concern was palpable.

Suspicions

Nowadays, attitudes about so-called "entitlement" can filter down into individual encounters. The major contact that many physicians have with disability is filing forms for patients anxious to obtain dispensation from the government or employers. Physicians tell me that this often makes them suspicious of patients' motivations. Certainly some patients do manipulate the system. However, suspicions are readily communicated nonverbally, especially to persons sensitized by embarrassment about their impairments. Judgmental disbelief is hurtful. Proving that what we experience is real can become a daunting task, as Mabel Bickford, an obese woman with bad knees who uses a wheelchair, said tearfully about talking to her physicians:

> "A lot of times I don't say anything, because if things get too out of control with my doctor, then emotionally I'm drained for the rest of the day. They just think that you don't *want* to walk. You just want to be in the wheelchair; it's comfortable. Well, you try it! I'm sure this plastic cuts my legs."

Being Invalidated

A common thread of failed communication is that persons with disabilities are somehow invalidated. In the most egregious instances, the invalidation is explicit, as suggested by two examples from medical school:

One day I encountered an attending physician, Dr. Winston, in a hospital lobby. "Hi, Lisa." he greeted me in a friendly way. "It's so good to see you." "Hello, Dr. Winston," I smiled.

"You always seem so cheerful when I see you," he said, pausing thoughtfully. "That must be one of the benefits of the inappropriate euphoria of MS. The inconvenience of MS is compensated by your always feeling happy. That must be why you are so generally pleasant."

That was definitely a conversation stopper. What did Dr. Winston mean? Any retort would be filtered through his faulty perceptions of my mental state and thus invalidated (for example, "She's just being overemotional—it's her MS"). This encounter raised a nagging doubt: are even my emotional stability and intellect under suspicion?

On my first day in the operating room during my surgical rotation, the attending surgeon let me hold a finger retractor during a delicate procedure. After the concentrated silence broke and closing began, the surgeon turned to me.

"What's the worst part of your disease?" he inquired.

Embarrassed by the assembled team of residents and nurses, I replied, "It's hard to talk about."

"Do you want my opinion?" he asked. The scrub nurse rolled her eyes at me empathetically. "You will make a *terrible* doctor," he continued. "You lack the most important quality of a good doctor: accessibility. You should limit yourself to pathology, radiology, or maybe anesthesiology." He turned to the anesthesiologist. "What do you think?" They planned my career.

Conversation in a Politically Correct Age

Finally, in the "politically correct" 1990s, disability has joined those topics in which language matters. Some disability advocates emphasize words, preferring, for example, "person who uses a wheelchair" to "wheelchair-bound patient." Although these preferences have solid rationales (for example, focusing on persons, not assistive devices), heightened semantic sensitivities undoubtedly chill some efforts at conversation with people who have disabilities. Our conversational partners are afraid of offending. Although I appreciate these difficulties, I believe they are quickly transcended by expressions of mutual respect and genuine interest, even if awkwardly phrased, and simple actions (for example, sitting down to be at the same eye level). As I suggest above, those of us with visible disabilities are conditioned to be "on guard."

The 1990 signing of the Americans with Disabilities Act brought the possibility that speech could convey discriminatory attitudes and presage actions that are now illegal. In retrospect, some positions expressed to me and actions taken during my four years in medical school (1980 to 1984) would probably be illegal under the Americans with Disabilities Act, which requires reasonable accommodations for persons with disabilities. For example, late in my third year, I began thinking about applying for an internal medicine residency. At a student dinner, I sat next to a leader at an affiliated teaching hospital, and I boldly asked his advice. I could not stay up all night, but few other accommodations seemed necessary.

"What would your hospital think of my situation?" I asked.

"Frankly," he replied in a conversational tone, "there are too many doctors in the country right now for us to worry about training handicapped physicians. If that means certain people get left by the wayside, that's too bad." There was silence around the table.

During the next months, I received little support from my medical school, and, after a wrenching internal debate (which was joined by my caring and realistic husband), decided to go straight into research.

I cannot imagine that anybody would say such things now as that hospital leader did in 1983. However, although legislation can regulate actions, it cannot control thoughts. Changing pervasive societal attitudes about persons with disabilities is clearly a long-term undertaking.

So, What Should I Say?

Communication is a two-way street. Both partners control—albeit sometimes unequally—conversational directions and outcomes. Therefore, my suggestions address persons on both sides of the issue.

For Persons with Disabilities

We should realize that many people have difficulty talking to us because of deeply embedded, complex emotions. Although overly simplistic, one explanation is certainly fear. Disability defines the one historically disadvantaged group that everyone can join in a flash. Perhaps the most obvious stigmata of disability is loss of control; this prospect terrifies Americans who are used to being in charge. One way to forestall this horrific possibility is to invalidate those who personify it.

Persons with disabilities constantly teach others about what our lives are like and, thus, what theirs may become. I take this educational role seriously, although I try to do it just by living my life. However, although it is desirable to aim for patience in frustrating situations, total equanimity is unrealistic. Sometimes people seem oblivious to the effect of their words or actions; saying something tart and corrective may vent our irritation and improve the situation (for example, motivate someone who is blocking our way to move). We must contend with being dismissed: "She's just upset because she's handicapped." Nonetheless, sometimes we should lighten up. Especially in casual contacts, one cannot alter deeply rooted attitudes. We frustrate ourselves rather than change minds.

Communication with physicians deserves special mention. Persons with disabilities, especially those progressively impaired by chronic illness, must talk directly to their physicians about their functional needs. For these patients, the discussion of acute concerns often consumes clinical encounters, and functional issues remain unaddressed. Certainly many physicians skillfully evaluate functional impairments and intercede to improve lives (for example, by prescribing physical therapy, assistive devices, or home modifications). Others, however, do not. Mrs. Jones described how her physician told her that she had MS:

> "The doctor spent about a minute and a half with me, and then he said, 'The bad news is, Mrs. Jones, you have MS. The good news is, when I saw you before, I wrote down three potential diagnoses in my notes. If you'd had either of the other two diagnoses, you would be dead by now.' Back then he never mentioned that to me. I said, 'Why didn't you tell me?' He said, 'The symptoms of the other diagnoses would have been so bad, you would've had to return, and I didn't want to upset you unnecessarily.' And with that, he left. He didn't tell me what to do. He didn't say, 'Do X.' He didn't say, 'Come back in six weeks.' He just left. Period. He spent about ten minutes, beginning to end. I was absolutely in shock."

Part of the problem is medical education. Many physicians know little about assessing and addressing functional problems. Until recently, most medical students were trained exclusively in in-patient settings, where acute illnesses or acute exacerbations of chronic disease are the focus. Nevertheless, another explanation is that physicians are people too. Physicians also experience fears, discomforts, and uncertainties about confronting disability that they cannot cure. In many instances, we must educate them.

For Persons without Disabilities

My first advice is to offer us choices and options. "Do you want help?" "How can we make things better for you?" Listen, and then respect our answers, even if they are a repeated, "No, thank you."

My second suggestion is for you to ask yourself: "Why does talking to this person make me uncomfortable?" This need not involve prolonged soul searching. The reasons will probably be obvious; potential solutions will readily follow. For example, many people tell me that they fear saying "the wrong thing." Acknowledge this fear openly: "Look, forgive me if I say something stupid." Remember that those of us with disabilities are awkward with words, too. We are often equally anxious to ensure productive communication.

Third, avoid doing what I did here—framing the argument as "us against them." I used this rhetorical device to explicate my arguments. Nonetheless, the well-worn phrase "we are all human," although trite, is true. The most visible feature that distinguishes you from me, perhaps, is my wheelchair. Each of us, however, carries private histories that differentiate us from all others; for some of us, only this one distinguishing feature is visible. For everyone, the joys and sorrows, hopes and fears that define our inner lives are invisible. Communication among people is always challenging for innumerable reasons. Identifying the role that disability plays is the first step in removing it from that complex mix of impediments.

Finally, if words and actions are obviously caring and respectful, communication will almost always be positive. For example, near the end of my first year of medical school, I was hospitalized briefly when I became completely unable to walk. Although I had tried to keep my situation secret, a classmate whom I barely knew came to my bedside one night.

"Gosh," he said reverentially, "I hear you have a really serious disease." The class had just learned about MS in neuropathophysiology.

"I guess so," I replied, uncertain what to add.

"Gosh." He paused again, obviously lost for words, but then he rallied. "I brought you cheesecake," he said. He handed me a big box and retreated hastily. When spoken with warmth, even awkward words are wonderful.

On Being a Patient: For Corrie

By Eric C. Last, D. O. (Doctorate of Osteopathic Medicine)

The birth of Corrie affected her parents in ways that no one anticipated. They were afraid that something was wrong with their baby soon after she was born. Later it was confirmed that Corrie has Down syndrome. After holding baby Corrie in their arms, her parents began to love and accept her just the way she is. The lives of Corrie's family have been changed in many ways; the entire family, including both sisters, watch Corrie's progress and new accomplishments with pride and affection. We cannot expect our lives to always remain the same. Unexpected joy or sorrow can happen to any of us anytime, providing new insights that can change our lives forever.

The birth of our third child was supposed to be a scheduled Cesarean section, performed at the hospital where I practice. However, several days before the appointed date, my wife began labor, and her scheduled section turned into an urgent one. Not long after the procedure began, our new baby, our Corrie, was handed to me with the pediatrician's pronouncement, "Here is your perfect baby girl." As I had done twice before, I cradled this new life in my hands, and tears of joy and thankfulness welled in my eyes. Too quickly, the circulating nurse took our new angel from me to be officially weighed and measured.

Not more than five minutes later, I felt a hand, gentle yet insistent, on my left shoulder. One of the nurses was there, whispering to me that the pediatrician needed to speak to me. I thought to myself that he was simply being a polite colleague, wanting to wish us luck. Nothing could be wrong, I reasoned, because he had used the words "perfect baby girl." But the look on his face as he waited for me in the hallway told me that something had changed. "I can't be sure," he began haltingly, "but I'm concerned that Corrie may have Down syndrome." He described "some things" that had him concerned, like very low muscle tone and a bothersome transverse crease on her palm. He told me about the tests that would be needed, the specialists who would be called. I shook his hand and thanked him for his thoroughness. I then felt a real physical pain, the likes of which I had never experienced in my life. It began in my gut, went up through my chest, and terminated in a wave of nausea and tremulousness that seized my entire being. I was helped to a chair, given a cup of water, and waited for the obstetrician to complete his work.

Fifteen minutes later, the obstetrician emerged from the OR, looking drawn and shocked. Someone had told him the events of the preceding minutes, and he immediately came to me and embraced me. Tears again welled up in my eyes, though now they were tears of grief and fear. Once composed, I asked how we were going to give the news to my wife. "That," he began slowly, "is something you are going to have to do." I tried in vain to get someone else to give her this piece of news, but all agreed it would be best handled by me.

I walked slowly toward the recovery room, the obstetrician's arm around my flagging shoulders. I recalled the many times I had given bad news to patients—news of cancer diagnosed, cancer recurred, AIDS, respiratory failure, any of the awful events that cause the body to fail. I wished I could be back in any of those situations, not to have to complete this task. I took a deep breath, entered the room, and held my wife's hand. "There might be a problem," I said clumsily. "The pediatrician thinks Corrie might have Down syndrome." My wife squeezed my hand, grimaced, and turned her head away. Within minutes, she was asleep again, momentarily escaping our new nightmare.

After spending a few moments in the delivery room lounge, trying to summon some strength, I somehow made my way downstairs to the doctor's lounge I had been in so many times before. I stared at the familiar phones, knowing I needed to pick one up and start dialing all the loved ones waiting anxiously to hear our good news. But the news I gave wouldn't be good. The hardest call was to our two older kids, telling them (with voice disguised as best I could) about their new sister, who was waiting to see them. I managed to complete the call, hang up the phone, and broke down again.

I returned to the nursery, where a pediatric geneticist was present, clipboard-toting assistant at his side, to catalog all of Corrie's parts. He rattled off a list of anomalies that were indicative of the presence of an extra chromosome. Yet, for each one, my brain jumped (ecstatically!) to another member who had a similar trait. And with each I became convinced that this was all an overreaction, doctors once again looking for things that weren't really there. Yet there was also a small voice in the back of my head reminding me about zebras and hoof beats. I knew that I didn't want to believe that something so awful, so strange, could be wrong with our child. Yet, I was starting to believe that they could be right.

The remainder of the first two days of Corrie's life was filled with new anxieties. There was difficulty obtaining blood for chromosome studies. Then there was the possibility of a cardiac problem, heralded by cyanosis whenever she cried. There were moments of solace, of comforting words, and positive thoughts from colleagues, perspective-building words from the social worker. But there was also a fellow physician who sank beneath insensitivity, gloatingly telling how his wife had an amniocentesis with each pregnancy. "Don't you know you could have terminated if she had an amnio," he asked. Don't you realize (I thought) you are talking about my very real, very alive baby?

Each day I wandered the hallways of the hospital, living each of Kubler-Ross's stages. Bargaining was the most interesting. I saw the pediatric ICU ambulance arrive from our affiliated teaching hospital. I thought how much nicer it would be if Corrie had an acute, life-threatening problem, where her future would hinge on some miracle of diagnostic acumen or surgical prowess, where the odds might be heavily stacked against her, but where her life would be forever normal if the procedure were a success. Instead, we had the possibility of a future filled with unknowns, and that unknown void would stretch out for the rest of Corrie's life and of ours.

Beyond the shock and fear, the overriding feeling during that first week was that something very special had been stolen from us. There were little things that should have happened but couldn't. The expectations of all the happy visits and handshakes in the hospital now turned into looks of sadness, expressions of condolence. There were walks to the nursery, gazing at all the newborns and staring at Corrie, trying to convince myself that she looked no different from the others. There was the traditional surf-and-turf dinner for new parents the night before discharge, when my wife and I went through the motions of enjoying ourselves, unable to hide our anxieties or sadness from each other.

One week after Corrie's birth, the geneticist called to say that yes, the results were in, and yes, there were three #21 chromosomes. But the real impact of that news didn't really hit until I saw the actual karyotype, with perfectly symmetrical rows of chromosome pairs, except above the number 21, where an extra piece of generic material lay waiting to change our family life forever.

It is now a year since Corrie's birth, and our lives truly have been changed, changed in ways I could not have imagined 12 months ago. No longer do I think of words like "horror" and "fear" when I describe our situation or her life. I think of the beautiful images I have seen: the joyful expression on my wife's face that has replaced her dread, the sheer delight our older children get when Corrie responds to their play, the look (that I'm convinced she reserves for me) Corrie gets when her daddy holds her, the incredible joy we all feel as she attains each milestone. I think of the progress she has made, and of the staff of teachers and therapists who have cared for her, and who have, for me, defined the word "dedication."

And yes, she has changed the way I live, and so has changed the way I practice medicine. I have a new sense of appreciation for my truly ill patients, and maybe a little less patience for those with trivial complaints. I have seen unbelievable coincidences in my practice, such as the friendship of a man I have cared for over the past six years, whose family has adopted a series of children with Down syndrome, or the grandmother who came into my office bursting with pride two years before Corrie's birth, telling me of her grandson's bar mitzvah, her grandson with Down syndrome. I have drawn strength from so many, including one patient, dying of AIDS, who knew of our situation and who cared enough to ask.

But mostly I think I have learned about myself and about love. And while we don't know what the future will hold for Corrie, I realize we can't predict this for anyone, even for ourselves. I realize I have made certain foolish assumptions in my life. I took it as a given that my children would all go to school, would all attain some stature in the world that I used to know and take for granted. But that world is very different to me now, and I realize just how arrogant such assumptions really are. And because of that, I have learned to try to appreciate all that surrounds me, as often as I can, for there is truly so much to be amazed by and to be thankful for.

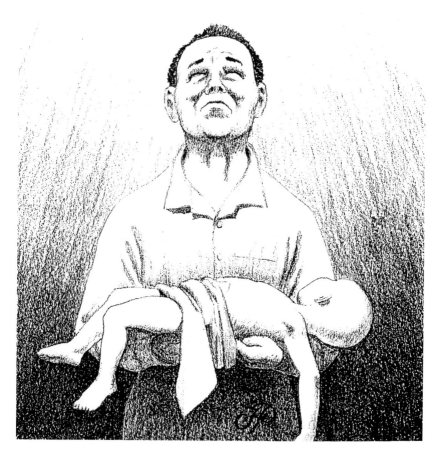

Illustrated by Herb Packard

"I think of Aaron and all that his life taught me, and I realize how much I have lost and how much I have gained. Yesterday seems less painful, and I am not afraid of tomorrow."

– Rabbi Harold S. Kushner

When Bad Things Happen to Good People

By Harold S. Kushner

Rabbi Harold Kushner shares his ordeal about the death of his young son, Aaron, and wonders where God is when you need him the most in his book When Bad Things Happen to Good People. *It is an attempt to make sense out of pain, suffering, and loss.*

Our son Aaron had just passed his third birthday when our daughter Ariel was born. Aaron was a bright and happy child, who before the age of two could identify a dozen different varieties of dinosaur and patiently explain to an adult that dinosaurs were extinct. My wife and I had been concerned about his health from the time he stopped gaining weight at the age of eight months, and from the time his hair started falling out after he turned one year old. Prominent doctors had seen him, had attached complicated names to his condition, and had assured us that he would grow to be very short but would be normal in all other ways. Just before our daughter's birth, we moved from New York to a suburb of Boston, where I became the rabbi of the local congregation. We discovered that the local pediatrician was doing research in problems of children's growth, and we introduced him to Aaron. Two months later—the day our daughter was born—he visited my wife in the hospital, and told us that our son's condition was called progeria, "rapid aging." He went on to say that Aaron would never grow beyond three feet in height, would have no hair on his head or body, would look like a little old man while still a child, and would die in his early teens.

How does one handle news like that? I was a young, inexperienced rabbi, not as familiar with the process of grief as I would come to be, and what I mostly felt that day was a deep, aching sense of unfairness. It didn't make sense. I had tried to do what was right in the sight of God. How could He do this to me?

Aaron died two days after his fourteenth birthday. This is his book—because his life made it possible, and because his death made it necessary.

I had gone beyond self-pity to the point of facing and accepting my son's death. A book telling people how much I hurt would not do anyone any good. This had to be a book that would affirm life. It would have to say that no one ever promised us a life free from pain and disappointment. The most anyone promised us was that we would not be alone in our pain, and that we would be able to draw upon a source outside ourselves for the strength and courage we would need to survive life's tragedies and life's unfairness. I am a more sensitive person, a more effective pastor, a more sensitive counselor because of Aaron's life and death than I would ever have been without it.

God, who neither causes nor prevents tragedies, helps by inspiring people to help. As a nineteenth-century Hasidic rabbi once put it, "Human beings are God's language." God shows His opposition to cancer and birth defects, not by eliminating them or making them happen only to bad people, but by summoning forth friends and neighbors to ease the burden and to fill the emptiness. We were sustained in Aaron's illness by people who made a point of showing that they cared and understood: the man who made Aaron a scaled-down tennis racquet suitable to his size; the woman who gave him a small handmade violin that was a family heirloom; the friend who got him a baseball autographed by the Red Sox; the children who overlooked his appearance and physical limitations to play stickball with him in the backyard and who wouldn't let him get away with anything special. People like that were "God's language"—His way of telling our family that we were not alone, not cast off.

In the same way, I firmly believe that Aaron served God's purposes, not by being sick or strange looking (there was no reason why God should have wanted that), but by facing up so bravely to his illness and to the problems caused by his appearance. I know that his friends and schoolmates were affected by his courage and by the way he managed to live a full life despite his limitations. And I know that people who knew our family were moved to handle the difficult times of their own lives with more hope and courage when they saw our example. I take these as instances of God moving people here on earth to help other people in need. And finally, to the person who asks, "What good is God? Who needs religion if these things happen to good people and bad people alike?" I would say that God may not prevent calamity, but He gives us the strength and perseverance to overcome it. Where else do we get these qualities which we did not have before?

Finding Hope & Compassion

Job's Story

Archibald MacLeish wrote a thought-provoking version of Job's biblical story in a modern setting that helps us to understand suffering. Even though Job was a good person, he was devastated by suffering and tragedy. Job's health fails, his children die, and his business fails. The city where Job lived is destroyed by an atomic bomb. In MacLeish's play, Job goes back to his wife, and they prepare to go on living together and building a new family. Their love, not God's generosity, will provide the new children to replace the ones who died.

Job forgives God and commits himself to go on living. His wife says to him, "You wanted justice, didn't you? There isn't any—there is only love." The two narrators, representing the perspectives of God and Satan, are baffled. How could a person who has suffered so much in life want more life?

MacLeish's Job answers the problem of human suffering, not with theology or psychology, but by choosing to go on living and creating new life. He forgives God for not making a more just universe, and decides to take it as it is. He stops looking for justice, for fairness in the world, and looks for love instead. In the play's moving last lines, Job's wife says:

The candles in church are out,
The stars have gone out in the sky.
Blow on the coal of the heart
And we'll see by and by.

The world is a cold, unfair place in which everything they held precious has been destroyed. But instead of giving up on this unfair world and life, instead of looking outward to churches or nature for answers, they look inward to their own capacities for loving. "Blow on the coal of the heart" for what little light and warmth we will be able to muster to sustain us.

Perhaps Love Is the Answer

Is there an answer to the question of why bad things happen to good people? That depends on what we mean by "answer." If we mean "is there an explanation which will make sense of it all?" then there is probably no satisfactory answer.

But the word "answer" can mean "response" as well as "explanation," and in that sense, there may well be a satisfying answer to the tragedies in our lives. The response would be Job's response in MacLeish's version of the biblical story—to forgive the world for not being perfect, to forgive God for not making a better world, to reach out to the people around us, and to go on living despite it all.

In the final analysis, the question of why bad things happen to good people translates itself into some very different questions, no longer asking why something happened, but asking how we will respond, what we intend to do now that it has happened.

Are you capable of forgiving and accepting in love a world which has disappointed you by not being perfect, a world in which there is so much unfairness and cruelty, disease and crime, earthquake and accident? Can you forgive its imperfections and love it because it is capable of containing great beauty and goodness, and because it is the only world we have?

Are you capable of forgiving and loving the people around you, even if they have hurt you and let you down by not being perfect? Can you forgive them and love them, because there aren't any perfect people around, and because the penalty for not being able to love imperfect people is condemning oneself to loneliness?

Are you capable of forgiving and loving God even when you have found out that He is not perfect, even when He has let you down and disappointed you by permitting bad luck and sickness and cruelty in His world, and permitting some of those things to happen to you? Can you learn to love and forgive Him despite His limitations as Job does, and as you once learned to forgive and love your parents even though they were not as wise, as strong, or as perfect as you needed them to be?

And if you can do these things, will you be able to recognize that the ability to forgive and the ability to love are the weapons God has given us to enable us to live fully, bravely, and meaningfully in this less-than-perfect world?

> "I think of Aaron and all that his life taught me, and I realize how much I have lost and how much I have gained. Yesterday seems less painful, and I am not afraid of tomorrow."

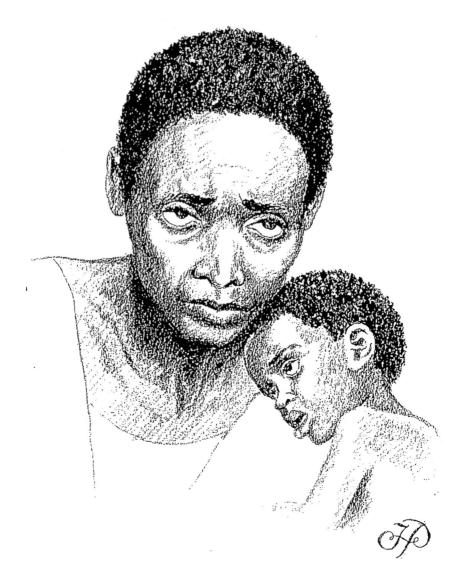

Illustrated by Herb Packard

"Who is going to care for my children?" "Who?" There are millions of orphans in Africa who have lost their parents to AIDS. These children face unbelievable grief in the future and may even have AIDS themselves.

I'm the Only One Left

By John Donnelly

The AIDS epidemic is worldwide. It ignores geographic and racial boundaries. Today new cases of HIV infection are mostly due to drug use by injection and heterosexual contact, but initially most cases in the United States were found in homosexual men.

The following excerpt is about disease in Malawi, a nation in southern Africa. AIDS has damaged the bodies of many people living there so that infectious diseases like tuberculosis, malaria, cholera, and bacterial meningitis are often fatal. Even when a correct diagnosis is made, the drugs to treat it may not be available. Poverty, malnutrition, and ignorance are everywhere.

Sounds echo through the concrete corridors of Lilongwe Central Hospital. Infants cry for their mothers, patients moan, nurses push squeaky carts. No sound is muffled until a scream silences everyone. It is a woman's scream, followed by another, and another. The sound seems to come from everywhere at once, and from nowhere. The woman pauses for a moment, and the buzz of the hospital fills the space. Then she finds her voice again. Her words are suddenly clear and close.

"Who is going to care for my children?" "Who?" "He didn't know he was going to die! He died on his way for X-rays!"

The small 20-year-old woman writhes and trembles on the second floor. She makes whooping sounds, she whimpers, she groans, and then goes quiet. Women sit around her, watching warily, afraid that she might flail her limbs at them.

Fifteen feet away, behind a door, three white-robed hospital attendants wearing disposable gloves carefully wrap a red-and-grey-checked woolen blanket around the body of her husband, Edson James, 42. He was a farmer. A storm of diseases took him; AIDS had demolished his body's defenses, turning ordinary germs into killers.

The attendants wrap rope around the blanket and knot it tight. They wheel the corpse into the hall on a gurney, the same one that served as the farmer's deathbed. As they wait for the elevator, they stare at the woman, who is face-down on the floor, now as still as her late husband. Five minutes have passed since her first scream. Everyone in the hallway looks at the bundle of death with new appreciation. From one corner, a nursing mother takes in the scene through hooded, dulled eyes. "Every two hours we expect someone to die here," says Priscilla Gunn, whose husband is a patient in another room. "Every hour we expect to hear cries."

The next morning, at 8 a.m., doctors, medical students, and the adult ward's head nurse walk into a small room on the hospital's third floor. It is time for their daily review of cases and deaths over the past 24 hours. Gift Mwalwanda Gumboh, the head nurse, appears calm. But she is very angry. "We had a fatal case yesterday of a man who was married to a very young girl," she tells her colleagues. "He came in a long time ago, and if we had 10 nurses on this ward, we would have noticed that he was failing. Instead we have one nurse for 78 patients! We decided to send him off for X-rays, and he died. The X-rays should have been done two weeks ago. The person was neglected. We need more personnel." It is a familiar story, another person passing away needlessly and almost unremarked. No one here takes the blame. Blame, they feel, should go to the system.

The morning meeting ends, and workers leave to check on patients. On the second floor alone are 98 patients waiting for one of three doctors or a half-dozen nurses. Fifteen medical students trail them.

We follow along, with our translator. She is Lisa Madsen, 24, who returned to Malawi earlier this year, leaving behind a life of possibility in London. She came back to care for her sister, who eventually died of AIDS, leaving behind three children. "I care for my nephew and nieces now," she says. "I'm one of six children, and I'm the only one left now. They all died of AIDS."

In a room down the hallway, meanwhile, two men carry in a new patient: Rebecca Makwenda, 26. It is 1:25 p.m. Rebecca is wheezing, lethargic, feverish, coughing. A doctor prescribes antibiotics and intravenous fluids. He leaves, and nurses insert the IV line into her withered right arm. At 2:15 p.m., a nurse checks on her. Rebecca is dead.

At the next morning's meeting, a student doctor reads from Rebecca's chart: "She had a headache for three weeks, diarrhea for three weeks. She developed a cough, had a fever, seemed chronically ill, had neck stiffness, possibly indicating meningitis. She likely had pneumonia. Diagnosis was sepsis, pneumonia, pulmonary TB, malaria."

It was not possible to say what killed her. AIDS weakened her immune system, and as many as five powerful diseases swept through her.

One doctor asks why she didn't come in earlier. No one has an answer. It is a question they ask almost every day.

The mortician is signing out the body of Rebecca Makwenda. Her husband, Henry Chirwa, a tall, thin, handsome man, a manager of a tobacco farm, waits patiently. He now has two children to raise by himself. A third child, Rose, died of pneumonia in June. She was one month old. With the help of relatives, Chirwa loads the casket carrying his wife into a pickup truck for the six-hour journey north, to her village of Tukombo. "My future," he says, "is bleak."

She was the third Makwenda sibling to die during the last year, possibly all from AIDS. Another had died two years earlier. The victims don't know how they were infected, although it was almost certainly through sexual contact. Although free AIDS testing is becoming widely available, the disease remains a largely unacknowledged killer because of the stigma it carries here and in other countries.

In the center of the village, under low-hanging mangoes, the church women stand erect in a circle around the casket, holding fistfuls of yellow flowers with their heads down. They also hold green bouquets woven into the shape of a cross. Church elders lift the casket onto their shoulders and trudge nearly a half-mile in the oppressive heat, until they reach the village cemetery.

Henry bends over the grave. "Rebecca, so dear to me," he whispers. "The family loved you. We are parting forever. We will never meet again. May your soul rest in peace."

The funeral is done. He must move on. One of Rebecca's brothers, Ephraim, is anxious to call a family meeting about Henry's and Rebecca's children. Ephraim, who lost his firstborn earlier in the year, wants to take care of Catherine, the youngest. "Let's put our mind to the children, what's best for the children," he tells Henry on the long walk back. Henry just stares ahead, saying nothing. When he arrives at the village, he walks away from his relatives and friends to a shady spot in a field. He says softly, so no one else will hear, "I want to keep my children. They're used to me. They're used to my voice."

He looks off in the distance. There's another issue. "The worst that can happen ..." He chokes up, then tries again. "The worst that can happen is maybe I'm infected, too, that I may go. I'm very worried." He must decide. Should he get tested for HIV? "I think of my kids' education, they are very young. I think I must know about myself," Henry says, his eyes fuzzy and bloodshot. "I think that's right." He turns and walks away. Henry Chirwa takes the HIV test. He is positive. He covers his face and weeps.

On Sunday, church comes to Lilongwe Central. Choirs enter the hospital all morning long, walk into rooms, surround beds, and burst out singing, their melodies echoing throughout the building. For many patients and workers, these are blessed moments. Some mouth the words. Some press their eyes closed, the better to take in the sounds. Life, for once, seems to fill these rooms, pressing death into the dark corners.

Death never leaves, though.

Robert and Shirley Hine

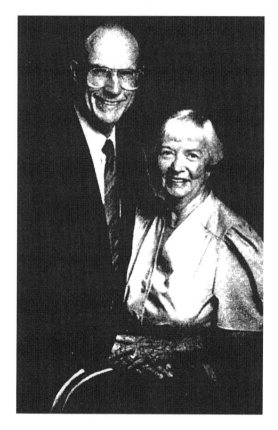

Author's photo

Taken during the year after surgery that restored Robert Hine's vision

Second Sight

By Robert V. Hine

Robert Hine gradually lost his eyesight starting at age twenty due to uveitis, an eye inflammation, a result of rheumatoid arthritis. Yet he became a distinguished history professor and wrote books about the early days of the American West. He became completely blind at age forty-nine when he developed cataracts in addition to the uveitis. Risky surgery for the removal of cataracts restored most of his vision after fifteen years of being blind. Robert describes his journey into darkness and return to the world of the sighted in his book, Second Sight.

I endured the first open news of blindness with a shrug. I was not that badly off. It was hard to feel sorry for myself. My eyes were only the tip of the iceberg. What I had really been fighting for years was a damnable case of juvenile rheumatoid arthritis. Huge bulbar, inflamed knees and elbows and wrists, in fact every joint, including my jaws, had stiffened and pained, and that lasted for years. I consumed salicylates like popcorn. I spent my seventeenth year immobilized in bed. The joints grew so locked that they had to be literally broken loose by husky therapists in a warm-water swimming pool. But so what? That was largely in the past, and who feels sorry for the past? The arthritis left me with an eye condition known as uveitis, more specifically, iridocyclitis. For both diseases, the doctors tried everything.

Initially, I thought my vision would improve and wrote in my journal, "I can say truthfully that my right eye has noticeably improved vision. Outlines are still very fuzzy, but objects can be distinguished with a fair amount of ease." However, three months later I wrote, "The old fiery redness and sandy discomfort, telltale signs of a uveitis flare-up, led me to board the bus down the Continental Divide for a medical look-see in Denver. That's where I got the black news." My vision was significantly impaired and I still had precipitates and active uveitis. When I looked back through my journal, I realized I was not only being unduly optimistic, but also unconsciously noting sounds more than sights. I was beginning my long descent into Arctic twilight. For me, the darkness did not crash down in some traumatic accident. It ate away like a shadow in the afternoon and led me to think that little was happening or at least the problem was not serious.

In the late 1950s Hine's ophthalmologist explained that cataracts were developing.

No one could say how fast they might grow; she would keep an eye on them. The cortisone was very likely causing the cataracts, but since the cortisone was thought to be and probably was keeping the uveitis at bay, and since uveitis itself could cause cataracts, treatment went on as before.

In 1967 I finished five years as chairman of the history department. Between then and 1970, the cataracts grew like hotbeds of spurge on a humid day. Vision dramatically clouded. During that time, layers of haze and floaters, swirls of lazily moving clots, became frenzied when I moved from light to darkness. If I were going blind from cataracts, why not surgically remove them? The cataract operation alone would not have been that big a deal. It was the uveitis that caused the hitch. That delicate condition would not take kindly to surgery.

In the 1960s, when my vision fell to a corrected 20/200 in the best eye, I was officially blind. But I did not accept the condition of blindness. I avoided the word. I was skillful in hiding the impairment from others and myself. With the white cane it was the same; there was reluctance and resistance. For years I did not use that badge of cowardice, when for safety I certainly should have.

In 1975, I fell down a flight of stairs and landed on gritty, pitiless brick. They were the steps to a party of friends. It was Thanksgiving time. I was in high spirits, with little thought of my blindness, which was pretty well advanced by then. After lots of help getting inside and a stiff drink, I was carted away in an ambulance, thereby completely spoiling the party. My hip was broken, requiring surgery, a pin, and months of recovery. Believe it or not, I still found excuses to avoid the white cane. However, after a second fall downstairs, I began using a cane cautiously. The general reluctance to use a white cane is only a symptom of the widespread hesitation to admit blindness.

No matter how I might try to be free, to write my own books, to deliver my own lectures, to provide for my own family, my daily life was the flip side of individualism. There is more than one technique, however, to writing history when blind, and I capitalized on at least three—Braille and recordings, live readers, and eventually talking computers. Braille was my basic salvation. My student readers were a pulsating joy. For my fifteen blind years, they sat across from me, averaging two or three a year, men and

Finding Hope & Compassion

women, freshmen and graduate students, conservatives and radicals, serious and lighthearted. I dedicated books to my readers, and I still have a list of their names that I cherish.

The blind must have order not chaos in their lives. Anything out of place is not only useless but does not exist. On the wrong table, the ashtray might as well be on Mars. I remember all too well the unwittingly moved glass; the coffee cup crashing to the floor; the misplaced notes never found. Thus the older person, or one who is by nature orderly, falls more easily into the familiar and the routine indispensable to sightlessness. It did not take me long to realize that anything not put where it belonged was chaotically lost and then to generalize that organization, like imagination, would give me at least half a chance to compete with the sighted. As John Hull put it, "Familiarity, predictability, the same objects, the same people, the same routes, the same movements of the hand to locate this or that—take these away, and the blind person is transported back into the infantile state where one simply does not know how to handle the world."

In 1986 the pressure in Robert's right eye rose above normal. The mature, ripe cataract was leaking, clogging up the system, and causing the pressure to build into secondary glaucoma. Emergency surgery restored most of his vision and included implantation of an intraocular lens. Right after the bandages were removed from his eyes, he looked about.

I turned to the one person I most wanted to see again, Shirley, and there was her silver hair shining, her loving face and eyes smiling. She did not seem changed to me. I guess I had been too close to her during those blind years to let her image slip away, rehearsing it with every joint experience, refusing to let her visually escape. After fifteen years, her face still glowed with that warm softness that I could see without touching. Now she was draped in color, wearing—was it deliberate?—a multi-colored blouse with wide stripes. I touched the colors and identified for her the yellow, the blue, the green. All the while my eyes looked over a new fairyland. The examination room was delightful—the counters of intense yellow, the bottles of clear glass and colored labels, the black-handled, silver-edged, glittering instruments.

Sight, of course, is not advantageous only to beauty; it is a tool of efficiency. I am impressed over and over at how much easier and more direct are my sighted efforts. I sweep now only that part of the walk that has leaves on it, not the whole walk. I move straight through a door, not pausing to feel for the edges. My hand reaches faster for the cup on the shelf, and I place the plug in the socket without fear and fumbling. Longhand multiplication no longer involves remembering all the figures in my head. The toothpaste goes directly onto the toothbrush (no longer on my tongue for measurement). The electric shaver stops clean-cut at the bottom of my sideburns. Most everything takes only one-half the time.

How many people have told me my second sight is a miracle? If what they mean is a blessing, there can be no doubt. I feel like Helen Keller, who invoked a sense of the miraculous when Anne Sullivan came into her life: "Thus I came up out of Egypt and stood before Sinai, and a power divine touched my spirit and gave it sight so that I beheld many wonders. And from the sacred mountain I heard a voice which said, *knowledge is love and light and vision.*" What might she have written had she regained her sight!

Robert Nutt

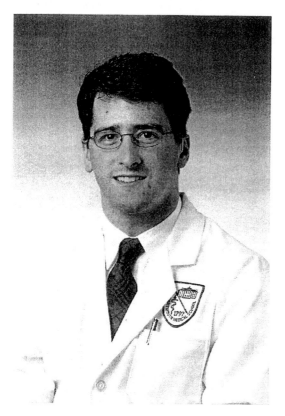

Photo by Mark L. Washburn

Silence Is Sound

By Rob Nutt

Rob Nutt is a Dartmouth medical student who lost his hearing as a child and then learned lip-reading and sign language. He wants to bridge the communication gap between the deaf and hearing, improving the quality of medical care for the deaf.

Profound changes are now sweeping the world of deaf children due to improved cochlear implants that are inserted into the ear by surgeons. Hearing and speech are markedly improved in almost all children who get implants before the age of four. Still, the debate over when to use implants is far from over. A child who is shown both oral and sign language has an opportunity to choose which world to live in.

"Robbie, why didn't you come when I…" My innocent expression stopped my mother from finishing. She lowered her voice and asked again without the rage. "Robbie, why didn't you come when I called you?"

"I didn't know you were calling me, Mom. Is dinner ready yet?" I stood up, taking my mother's hand, and followed her down the stairs where dinner was waiting. We had been through this before, but now my mother realized that this might not be simply a phase that I was going through.

I was not yet four years old at the time. It was the spring before kindergarten and my mother had just had her third child. Whether or not my mother or I was aware of it, this was also the day that we first knew I was deaf. Over the next several months I went through a number of tests. I can remember my first audiogram at the Children's Hospital of Philadelphia like it was yesterday.

I remember the nurse. As we walked through the halls, her face was the only thing that comforted me other than my mother's hand and my thumb (which was more often in my mouth than not). When I got to the testing booth, it all felt so familiar. There were stuffed animals, more than I had ever seen! Before shutting the door, the nurse explained the game I was going to play. I would raise my hand every time I heard a beep in either ear and then the animals would spin and clap. She placed the headphones on my head and smiled before closing me in.

The first time I heard a beep, I raised my hand, just as the nurse had told me. I flinched when suddenly all the animals began spinning and clapping. My head spun around when I looked back through the window in front of me. I probably had no idea why I was trapped in that box or why I was raising my hand, but I was having fun. The stuffed animals were my friends.

I was so scared that I must not have said a single word the whole time I was in that hospital. They had probably concluded that I was losing my hearing even before they locked me in the booth, since I was four years old and couldn't speak! Still, I do not look back on that day with any kind of anger. It was an adventure for me, and my mother's face never showed any sign that she was going to love me less if I couldn't make the animals spin and clap as many times as I was supposed to. As far back as I can remember, my parents never showed any sign of neglect, guilt, anger, or shame because their son did not have normal hearing. In fact, it is much more complicated than what my parents did or did not express.

Life itself is challenging and complicated, and being deaf has made it much more complex. Both my parents have continuously done everything they can to help me deal with the demands and expectations of a world that depends so much on sound. And when they cannot do anything for me, they support me in such a way that has made my friends admire the relationship I have with them.

My hearing loss began when I was a child and became worse as I grew older. I have been asked by a number of my friends, especially those who are deaf, if I have ever thought about what it would have been like had I gone to a deaf school to learn sign language when I was younger as opposed to being mainstreamed in a hearing community which requires lip-reading. Indeed, I have thought about it, but to be angry with my parents for not putting me in a deaf school when I was younger would be ridiculous. Whether or not it was the best thing for me to be sent to Chestnut Hill Academy as opposed to Pennsylvania School for the Deaf (PSD) or Clarke School is of little significance, especially at this point in my life after I have accomplished so much.

Helen Keller once said, "So much has been given to me, I have no time to ponder that which has been denied." This quote is cherished by the deaf community. There is time for frustration and anger, but my past defines who I am and to deny it would be an outright rejection of myself. How could I be angry with my parents for trying to find that school where I would learn to cope with whatever life should throw my way?

Although mainstreaming has defined my education, there are three paths that I have had a chance to choose from, overall. One is that of a deaf person, dependent on sign language and perhaps limited by silence. Then there is that of a deaf person who is an oralist struggling with lip-reading in the unfamiliar world of the hearing. The path that I have chosen is a combination of both sign use and speaking with the help of lip-reading in the deaf and hearing worlds. This requires balance and the will to experience the frustrations of both the deaf and hearing. Because I have chosen this path and not the others, my life has become particularly challenging and complex.

The years between third and eighth grade are a challenging period for me to recall or even write about. Looking back, it seems that those years were much lonelier than I was aware of at the time. It seemed to me that I was just like everyone else. I had not yet completely accepted my deafness, for I was not fully aware of the impact it was having on me.

Since my hearing loss is progressive, there was never anything constant that I could adjust to; my hearing would be different a month or two down the road. The impact this had on my communication affected the interactions I had with my surroundings, including my family. It was difficult for me to establish a sense of security within myself and with the world around me. I went into a state of denial; I tried so hard to be like everyone else. Although this behavior is typical of any adolescent, relative to my peers, my reasons were unique.

As I lost more of my hearing, I began to rely more on reading lips. Because of the impossibility of reading more than one set of lips at a time, group situations became very difficult for me. For instance, I found myself laughing just because others were laughing and not because I found something humorous. When it came to groups, I learned to value people's company over their words. It made me so happy to be invited out with a group that the fact that I couldn't hear everything did not matter so much anymore. This was a time when I was in denial. It hurts to admit it now because it makes me wonder how much I am still a prisoner of this effort to immerse myself with those who can hear.

While group situations continued to be a challenge for me, I did not let them keep me at home. I took advantage of other parts of my character that attracted people to me. Socially, especially among teenagers, smaller groups tend to be more intimate. It is during these gatherings that kids share their innermost questions, experiences, and feelings. We contribute and listen to conversations about dating, alcohol, personal experiences with peers, and other forms of general information. The fact that I watched the lips of whoever was talking did several things. First, it made the speaker feel that someone was listening to them. It also showed I was interested in what they had to say, which is something every person wants. Unfortunately, my attentiveness was often misinterpreted. On several occasions, the girl I was listening to interpreted this as an act of affection. I cannot say that I never followed through, but it is funny to some degree that my lip-reading adds a different tone to the conversation!

After my freshman year in college, I visited a psychologist who explained my situation metaphorically. It was late at night and the lights in his office were dimmed. I sat across from him and listened. I had never felt that a hearing person, no matter how educated, could understand my experiences, but by this time I was desperate, and so I listened to his words. "Rob," he said sitting up in his large leather chair, "you are standing in the middle of a circle of flames and if you do not find a way of controlling them, they will engulf you—you will be burnt." I had my doubts that this man understood my situations, and yet he created an accurate image of my anger and frustration. In order to survive, I must control emotional outbursts that can surround and attack me from any direction like fire whose depth lacks any form or consistency. I can feel the heat grow when I turn toward the flames. To this day, I have been searching for ways to dance calmly in the circle without yelling "Fire" when under stress.

I added manual communication to my bag of skills in eighth grade. My parents never prohibited me from learning sign language and I am not sure why I decided to learn sign then. I realized that one day I would be alone at college and since my hearing loss is progressive, I feared awaking to find my residual hearing gone. And so I decided to learn a language that I had heard of years before, a language that does not rely on sound. Sign language made it easier for me to meet other deaf people, but it also made my identity crisis even more difficult. I couldn't try to be like everyone else anymore.

Taking up sign language was a big step in accepting my deaf side.

During my senior year in high school, I taught eighth graders at Pennsylvania School for the Deaf for my Senior Project, an unpaid internship for seniors during their last month of high school. Traveling between a world dependent on sounds for communication and the other dependent on sight was like a daily commute between New York and Paris. I found it easy to communicate since my only limitation was learning more sign. It made me wonder why I had subjected myself to the struggle of being main-streamed.

Mrs. Dona Marler, my project advisor, helped me realize all that I had accomplished as a result of dealing with my challenges. Somehow she convinced me that being able to live in both the hearing world and the deaf world is a gift. I am in a unique position to bring the deaf community and hearing mainstream closer together. The degree of my hearing loss and my interpersonal skills allow me to interact effectively with both those who hear and those who do not. Although "living on the fence" is difficult, it has allowed me to contribute more by bridging the gap between the Hearing and the Deaf. This lesson came during a time when I was considering career alternatives to the perplexing issues that my physician father described when he came home from the hospital each night. Medicine became my homing beacon, a profession where I would be able to integrate my personal and academic interests with my determination to help others, the deaf community in particular. I will have the opportunity to teach my medical colleagues about the importance of being able to communicate well with patients and peers. One specific way that I could facilitate this is to help the medical community understand the deaf community. It has been pointed out to me that while teaching American Sign Language classes, I not only teach my students how to communicate with their hands, but I also teach them how to express their thoughts more effectively—with precision, patience, endurance, and a sense of humor.

During my sophomore year in college, Kathleen Dameo-Beatty, a deaf representative from Gallaudet University, spoke at the Association of American Medical Colleges conference on the issue of medical students with disabilities. In particular, she addressed the topic of hearing impairments and pointed out that there is a need for deaf doctors. My initial reaction to this was skepticism. I knew that medicine was the field that intrigued me, but at the time, my hearing loss had little significance on my decision to become a physician. When I asked my deaf friends and their families if it would make any difference for the deaf community to have a deaf physician, they felt it would be a much-needed improvement. I see myself being in a position to answer this need at least in that community where I practice medicine.

My thoughts about cultural barriers in health care were confirmed when I read an article in the *New York Times* entitled, "Language Barriers Are Hindering Health Care" (November 23, 1997). The article addressed cultural and linguistic frustrations that have developed between non-English-speaking patients and their doctors. It may be adequate for a deaf individual to come into the ER and be taken care of with the help of an interpreter; however, there seems to be a need for a deeper, more comfortable and trusting relationship between members of the deaf community and their personal physician. As a deaf doctor, I will make myself accessible to deaf individuals who will find a more comfortable and efficient avenue for medical care.

Since beginning medical school, my life's challenges have only intensified. I have had encounters with physicians who, upon learning of my hearing loss, question whether I should be here. With the help of engineers, I have designed and developed my own stethoscope and another device for the operating room; I struggle to get classmates to keep their hands away from their mouths and not mumble so that I can understand conversation. Some have come a long way; many still don't understand. I have my handful of friends whom I can confide in when things get to be overwhelming. One cold winter afternoon, while talking to one such friend, I had one of those moments when everything becomes clearer. In the course of a long conversation at the end of a particularly challenging day, I said to her, "I am going through a system that is not set up for me, and yet I continue through it because it is what is required of me if I want to become what I have always dreamed of becoming."

She replied, "But Rob, isn't that the story of your life?"

Throughout my struggles, I keep in mind the following poem. It contains lessons for all.

Finding Hope & Compassion

Listen

Author Unknown

When I ask you to listen to me
and you start giving me advice,
you have not done what I asked.

When I ask you to listen to me
and you begin to tell me why
I shouldn't feel that way,
you are trampling on my feelings.

When I ask you to listen to me
and you feel you have to do something
to solve my problem,
you have failed me,
strange as that may seem.

Listen! All I asked was that you listen,
not to talk or do—just hear me.
Advice is cheap;
Twenty cents will get you both
Dear Abby and Billy Graham
in the same newspaper.

And I can do for myself.
I am not helpless.
Maybe discouraged and faltering,
but not helpless.

When you do something for me
that I can and need to do for myself,
you contribute to my fear
and inadequacy.

But when you accept for a simple fact
that I do what I feel,

no matter how irrational,
then I can quit trying to convince you
and can get about this business
of understanding what's behind
this irrational feeling.

And when that's clear,
the answers are obvious
and I don't need advice.
Irrational feelings make sense when
we understand what's behind them.

Perhaps that's why prayer works,
sometimes, for people—
because God is mute
and He doesn't give advice
or try to fix things.

He just listens
and lets you work it out for yourself.
So please listen and just hear me.
And if you want to talk,
wait a minute for your turn—
I'll listen to you.

Constance Brinckerhoff

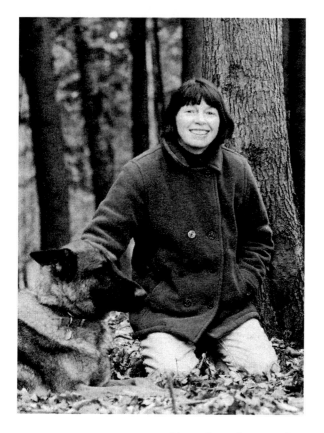

Photo by John Douglas

The Winter of Our Discontent

By Constance Brinckerhoff, Ph.D.

"Now is the winter of our discontent made glorious summer by the sun of York." —William Shakespeare, *King Richard III*

In this article from Dartmouth Medicine, *Dr. Brinckerhoff describes her battle against breast cancer in a way that she hopes will prove helpful to others fighting similar battles. Constance and her husband, Robert, enjoy walking their dogs through the wintertime woods. Giving their dogs daily walks helped her find courage and comfort throughout her cancer treatments. However, she cautions others that her normal strength did not return until a year after her treatments had been completed.*

Dr. Brinckerhoff is the Nathan Smith Professor of Medicine and of Biochemistry and the Associate Dean for Science Education at Dartmouth Medical School. She has also served as acting provost of Dartmouth College.

On June 6, 1996 my sister died of breast cancer at Dartmouth-Hitchcock Medical Center. She had lived with her disease for eight years, and about 18 months before her death she had moved to Norwich, Vermont, to be near my husband and me. We helped to care for her, but despite the excellent treatment she got here, her disease was too advanced. I watched her slowly decline and finally die. She was, literally, eaten alive by the cancer.

One week later, I went for my own yearly mammogram. My appointment was for 8:30 a.m., and I figured that I would be at work in the lab by 9:15. The technician did the manual exam quickly and thoroughly; in fact; she did such an excellent job that I remember complimenting her on her skill. Then she took the films, and I figured I was nearly done.

But she returned to the exam room a minute later, saying she wanted to take another film of one breast. I began to feel just a bit anxious; had I shifted as that image was taken?

It turned out the problem was not so simple. The technician guided my hand to my left breast and asked if I felt a lump.

"I guess so," I said.

"For how long?" the technician asked.

"I had no idea. I just thought it was normal…" My voice trailed off as the full meaning of the question sank in.

Within a few minutes, I was led down the hall for an ultrasound. There it was: a black hole in my left breast, about a centimeter in diameter—a little more than half an inch. "Suspicious," but not definitely malignant, I was told. I needed a cutting-needle biopsy, which was suddenly scheduled for 2:00 p.m. that same afternoon, Thursday, June 13. I left the hospital in a daze, my heart pounding. How could this be happening to me? I felt as though I had stumbled into a terrible soap opera script.

Instead of going to work, I went home, where my husband was. I told him the news. That afternoon we went back to DHMC for the biopsy. Although the doctor said there was only a 20 percent chance that the lump was malignant, his voice told me otherwise. He knew. Experience told him. The resident said, "Good luck" as she left the room.

I *knew* it was cancer.

On Friday, the 14th, I found out that, indeed, it was. Although the circumstances surrounding the acquisition of this knowledge differ for every woman with breast cancer, and, in fact, for everyone who ever receives a diagnosis of cancer, this moment is one of shared experience. There is a whole array of emotions, all mixed up together: disbelief, fear, shock, confusion, numbness. In an instant, your world is turned upside down, and no matter what follows it will never again be exactly the same.

My surgery was scheduled for the following Monday. I was lucky: the tumor was small and I could have a lumpectomy, along with the standard lymph node dissection. After the operation, the surgeon told me that all had gone very well: he got clean margins, and the nodes looked good. Whew! It looked like I would have just a brush with this disease and then could get on with my life. I was, after all, still trying to assimilate my sister's death barely a week earlier.

On Wednesday morning, my brother sent me a dozen beautiful pink roses. They were lovely, and I was recovering nicely from surgery. I felt happy and confident. Then the phone rang, and on the other end was the surgeon, telling me that the pathology report had come back and it turned out that I had one positive lymph node.

"The train has left the station…"

"The horse is out of the barn…"

Whatever metaphor I used to cloak it, the fact was that the disease had spread, at least at a microscopic level. Chemotherapy was called for, and that terrified me.

I knew that tumor cells do not, thank goodness, divide as fast in the body as they do in the lab. I knew that I had a little time to try to get used to the idea of what I was facing. I had just watched my sister die from the disease, and then, one week later, received the same diagnosis. I decided to put the chemo off until the end of the summer, hoping to enjoy the sun and regain some sense of equilibrium.

I truly was terrified of chemotherapy. I had always prided myself on being prepared, but I was at a loss to know how to prepare for what I was now facing. I talked with women who had gone through it. Each of them had a story of tremendous personal courage. They were all wonderful: caring, empathetic, warm, supportive. "It's not too bad," many of them said. I remained terrified.

Finally, at the end of August, the day of my first treatment came. My oncologist had suggested that I get six high-dose infusions, with three weeks between each treatment—meaning that I would be done by Christmas. Wonderful. It would all be over in a flash. But the reality was that time seemed to stand still, and my white counts never recovered sufficiently to make a three-week cycle possible. It was always four weeks.

The fall and winter dragged on. I began to relish those few days of each month when I would feel almost human, right before they "infused" me again.

But then, somewhere in the middle of it all, I learned that I *could do* what I had been dreading so much. I *could* hope. It was an enormous feeling of personal triumph. In the lab, we wrote five papers during the six months that I was on chemo. I walked the dogs a mile and a half every day during that time, with but two exceptions. I always felt better after the walk. Some structure, some goals, were important, I found. But I was clearly not myself. I was getting a CMF regimen, rather than CAF, which meant that all my hair would not fall out, although it thinned considerably and what was left had no life.

But I considered myself lucky—I still had some hair. Nonetheless, I coined a new term: a "dead hair day."

Chemo ended. Radiation began. It took 20 seconds, every day, Monday through Friday, for six and a half weeks. Sounds like nothing—20 seconds. Everyone told me it would be a "piece of cake." Not so. I got tired. I also got some type of radiation burn. One chilly March morning I actually walked the dogs with my chest bared, just to feel the cool air on my skin.

Finally, on April 14, ten months to the day after my diagnosis, I finished my therapies. As I got off the table in the radiation therapy room, I suddenly burst into tears. I am certain I was not the first nor would I be the last patient to do that.

What did I learn? How did those months change my life? First, although the diagnosis of cancer is scary, it is also somewhat remote, at least with early-stage breast cancer. You feel fine. There are no symptoms, no phenotype. For me, it was the *treatments* that taught me. They were very hard physically. But from them I learned to confront the possibility of my own mortality, an exercise that I had previously thought to be reserved for "others." The experience has made me stronger emotionally and more confident. It has also given me a perspective on what is really important. Where do I want to place my energies? I have also realized that cancer is not the only traumatic event that befalls people; life's difficulties come in many dark colors and breast cancer is only one of them.

Most of all, I have learned that I am very, very lucky. My disease was caught early. I have had exceptional medical treatment and emotional support, from physicians, friends and family, especially my husband. Spouses are a singularly unrecognized partner in this ordeal of breast cancer. As hard as it is for the patient to deal with the effects of treatment, it is also hard for those around us to see someone they know and love transformed from a normally energetic and enthusiastic individual into a creature curled up in the fetal position, or struggling to just put one foot in front of the other.

So then it was over, right? Life got back to normal, right?

Wrong. Where was my energy? Why was I still so very tired? Many people, including me, wondered why I was not resuming my full schedule. Rest, rest, rest: that seemed to be all that I was capable of some days. But finally, imperceptibly, about six months after I had finished my treatments, I was almost back to "normal." It was a full year, however, before I was truly myself again.

At the time of my diagnosis and during my treatments, I received tremendous support from other women who had had breast cancer. One, who was two years "out," assured me that she was fine, doing very well in fact, and that she was waiting for me to join her "on the other side." At the time, this phrase had no meaning for me. I could not comprehend any reality other than that of cancer, chemo, and radiation. But now I, too, am two years "out" and am "on the other side."

Today, there is no evidence of disease in my body, although I know that the jury will be out on the question for at least another three to five years. Tumor cells are tricky little buggers, and they can, if they want, change and mutate in response to the pressures that are put on them—and pop up again in some other part of the body.

Ironically, just about the time of my diagnosis, my research laboratory began studying breast cancer. In contrast to many investigators who are studying why the cells divide abnormally, or what genes are responsible for breast cancer in the first place, we are studying how the cells break away from their original home in the breast, jump onto the highways that are our blood vessels and lymph channels, and travel to other parts of the body. It is, after all, the tumors that metastasize to vital organs such as the liver, lung, and brain that kill—not the original tumor in the breast. Can we block this travel? Can we prevent the tumor from colonizing elsewhere in the body?

As I go about my life now, days will pass without my even thinking about the fact that I have had breast cancer. My life is full, productive, and happy. I am taking tamoxifen, with no apparent side effects. I am grateful not only for its anticancer benefits, but also for the estrogen-like effects it has on bones and the cardiovascular system. My regular checkups at DHMC offer an opportunity to visit with good physicians who are also friends and colleagues.

No one can tell me for sure what the future will bring, but I hope I am prepared for whatever lies ahead. I have been privileged throughout this experience to meet many terrific women with the disease. Their stories are full of courage, many far more than mine. What I tell others who are where I was two years ago is that my own journey through those ten months was very, very hard—but it was not "bad."

"In the midst of winter, I finally learned that there was in me an invincible summer." —Albert Camus

Tom and Peggy Gilbert

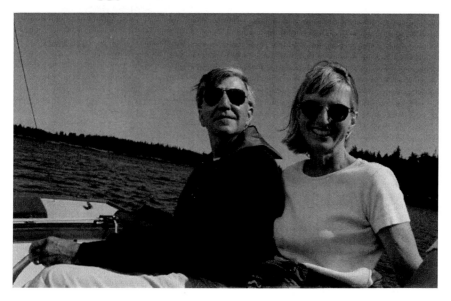

Author's photo

Sailing on their boat *Patience* off the coast of North Haven, Maine, one year after Tom's stroke.

The Impact of a Stroke on a Marriage

By Peggy Gilbert

Thomas Gilbert is a graduate of Dartmouth Medical School, Class of 1972, and a highly respected family physician. His wife Peggy is a college counselor. Tom's stroke has deepened their love and helped them to find new meaning and direction in their lives in spite of the dramatic changes caused by Tom's stroke.

"Why isn't Tom coming down to the dock?" I wondered. We were on vacation in North Haven, Maine, and I was surprised that Tom, who is an avid sailor, was nowhere in sight. Eventually, I found him disoriented and lying in bed. One minute he had been an active doctor, husband, father, friend; the next he was a helpless fifty-two-year-old stroke victim. A CAT scan at Penobscot Bay Medical Center determined that the stroke was caused by a massive hemorrhage on the left side of his brain. The neurologist told me that Tom needed to be moved to a major medical center immediately, and that he would either die or be permanently disabled. He was flown by helicopter to Massachusetts General Hospital.

It was a huge shock to see my husband so disabled. Occasionally his facial expressions reminded me of the "real" Tom, but mostly he was hidden beneath a stroke-induced fog. I wanted to crawl into the ICU bed with him and have him put his arm around me and tell me that everything would be okay, but he was in a deep coma and hooked up to every machine imaginable. In an effort to remind the doctors, nurses (and ourselves!) that this comatose patient had recently led a vibrant, meaningful life, our family brought in pictures from home to display around the room.

Periodically, the doctors and nurses would ask Tom his name, where he was, and to hold up two fingers. Eager for their father to respond correctly, Carrie and Dan (ages 24 and 23, respectively) would demonstrate what he was supposed to do. But Tom was unable to follow a simple command. He couldn't speak, and we were not certain that he knew who we were or understood what we were saying. When he was transferred to Spaulding Rehabilitation Hospital, his body was as floppy as a rag doll. It took two physical therapists to get him into an upright position, and he became exhausted after sitting up for short periods. I wondered if our life would ever be normal again.

Until Tom's stroke, I had never felt extreme despair. I remember sitting in my car in the parking lot at the school where I worked and reciting St. Francis of Assisi's prayer, "Make Me an Instrument of Thy Peace," hoping that God would give me the strength and courage to get through the day. When I left Tom in his hospital room at the end of the day, I was so exhausted and discouraged that I felt numb. Walking to my car, I felt defeated and alone.

I was surprised that none of the attending physicians talked with our family about our feelings of despair and anxiety. That task was delegated to a lovely, young social worker who stopped by periodically. Our son commented that the medical residents resembled packs of dogs as they raced from patient to patient, avoiding eye contact with the families. The neurosurgeon who spent six hours removing the cavernous malformation of vessels from Tom's brain did not come down to the family waiting room to discuss the outcome of the procedure. Instead, I was directed to a phone booth where we had a brief conversation. I remember telling a colleague at work that I had met some extraordinary technicians, but had not yet interacted with a physician who seemed wise.

Fortunately, our family, friends and colleagues provided lots of support. Our daughter Carrie, who is a marathon runner, encouraged me to exercise to release tension. I discovered that I do feel better after biking, swimming, or lifting weights and began exercising on a regular basis. Our son Dan, who was living in San Francisco, moved back to Boston so that he could actively participate in Tom's recovery. Before he moved east, he wrote us beautiful letters that often included an inspirational quote from Martin Luther King, Shakespeare or Bob Dylan. Knowing that Dan believed that we could survive this crisis gave me courage to persevere. He set up an e-mail account where friends could get periodic updates on Tom's progress. Many wrote wonderful messages to Tom full of fond memories and hope for the future or shared stories of personal suffering, giving us perspective on our situation. Carrie would print out the messages at work and read them to Tom while he ate his dinner in his hospital room. His obvious pleasure in this nightly ritual was one of the first signs that his comprehension was intact. Several dear friends visited Tom on a regular basis, reading to him, joking with him and generally cheering him (and us!) on. A former colleague of Tom's sent us tapes of his favorite folk and operatic music. Although I do not understand Italian, Pavarotti's plaintive aria helped me cry.

At the time of Tom's discharge from the hospital, I wasn't convinced that I was capable of caring for him. After all, he had a team of skilled therapists, nurses and doctors in the hospital, and there was only me at home. I voiced my concerns to his hospital team, and they assured me that we would do just fine. Upon his arrival in Millis, Tom wanted to get out of his wheelchair and go for a walk. I had been taught how to shadow him so I dutifully held onto his belt as he wandered around our yard. Periodically, I would remind him that he should rest, but he insisted on continuing. Then he stumbled and started to fall. I couldn't stop his fall (but I managed to slow it down), and I couldn't pick him up. Used to being in control, I found it very difficult to call 911. I felt like a huge failure. The kind officer reminded me that it is okay to ask for help.

I began meeting with a social worker to discuss my reactions to Tom's stroke. "So tell me, when did your world turn upside down?" she asked. It was an enormous relief to have someone acknowledge all the changes in my life. I had resigned from my job to care for Tom and was feeling isolated and lonely at home. Instead of an equal partnership with my husband, I was now "in charge." In some respects, I felt more like a parent than a wife. My tendency was to be overprotective (especially after his fall and the 911 call), but gradually I began to relax and to "let go." Clearly Tom was happier when he was able to do things for himself. I'll never forget the grin on his face the day I returned from an errand to discover that he had dragged the ladder from the garage and filled the bird feeders.

Like many others who have had a stroke on the left side of the brain, Tom has aphasia, or difficulty speaking and writing. When he first came home from the hospital, our "conversations" resembled the game of Twenty Questions in that often I had to ask him "yes" and "no" questions to figure out what he meant. Because it was such an effort, we didn't talk a lot and our home was eerily quiet. While the phone and e-mail enabled me to interact with others, I felt guilty chatting with friends while Tom sat isolated in his wheelchair. Prior to his stroke, he had been the computer whiz in our home. After the stroke, he couldn't remember how to turn on the computer or even spell his name. Slowly but surely, month by month, Tom has made tremendous strides. The pace of his speech is slower, and he cannot always recall the exact word he wants, but he usually communicates effectively. Our most meaningful conversations occur when we are both relaxed; our worst are when I try to speed things up by finishing his sentences. His writing is improving as well. Now he writes short e-mail messages.

Recognizing that I am an extrovert who is energized by interactions with others, "my" social worker/counselor encouraged me to reconnect with friends and colleagues and to think about returning to work eventually. At her suggestion, I called a member of our Aphasia Support Group whom I had admired at the monthly meetings to ask if she would meet me for coffee. I was feeling particularly down and wondered if Tom and I would ever be truly happy again. Not only did she meet with me, she invited Tom and me to dinner later that week so that we could get a feel for how she and her husband had managed during the seventeen years since his stroke. That evening was a turning point for me. I saw that one does not have to devote all one's time to one's spouse's recovery. In fact, Tom's and my future happiness might depend on our having somewhat separate lives, just as we did prior to his stroke.

Perhaps because Tom is a family physician, I feel a mixture of sadness and comfort when we meet with our family doctor. Sadness that Tom is no longer practicing medicine and comfort that I am meeting with a doctor who, like Tom, is both smart and kind. He listened to our concern that Tom's anti-seizure drug was making him groggy and came up with a plan to wean Tom off the medication. When Tom's neurosurgeon postponed an appointment to review some important tests, he made time to interpret the results for us. While we don't call him frequently, he always returns our phone calls promptly. He encourages Tom to report his progress with his speech, occupational and physical therapy, even though it would be more efficient for me to summarize. He has been open to our exploring alternative therapies such as hypnosis. In this age of managed care and fifteen-minute appointments, I feel blessed to have a compassionate physician who listens carefully and offers meaningful advice. I have met with him individually on several occasions to talk about my deep sense of loss. We have talked about the difference between depression and grief, and he has encouraged me to grieve. We have also discussed the fact that family members grieve at different points. At this point, Tom's focus is on recovery.

Over the Memorial Day weekend and nine months post-stroke, Tom and I visited the cemetery where his parents are buried. Seeing Tom walking with a cane toward their grave made me cry. "It would break their hearts to see you like this," I told him. "Yes, if they compared me to a year ago. But don't you think they would be proud of all the progress I've made since the stroke?" he replied. He had a point. No longer unsteady on his feet, he routinely walks a mile or more each day with the assistance of his cane. He has learned to swim again. I tease him that he looks like an otter as he glides up and down the pool on his back with his affected arm resting on his belly. He drives a car with a left foot pedal and passed his driver's license. Since his right arm and leg remain paralyzed, every movement requires extraordinary concentration, effort and time. If I ask Tom a question when he is walking down stairs or getting dressed, he gets irritated and asks me to wait until he is finished. Prior to his stroke, Tom and I allowed an hour to get ready for work each morning; now we assume that it will take two hours for him to bathe, get dressed and eat.

After ten months of inpatient and outpatient therapy, where we received invaluable help from many dedicated professionals, Tom exhausted both his health plan benefit package and himself. In need of a break, we returned to North Haven where our saga began. Life is so ironic; never have we had so much time on this idyllic Maine island, yet now we are limited in what we can do. In past years, Tom would spend every free minute messing around in boats. Now he is dependent on my help to get him from our dock to the boats. His biggest challenge is getting in and out of our rowboat. First he kneels down, and then he lies flat on his back and scoots over to the edge of the dock, where he swings his legs into an inflatable dinghy. Finally, he gets into a sitting position and uses his "good" arm to lift his body and push himself into the boat. Meanwhile, I am holding the boat stable and praying that he won't lose his balance. The whole process probably takes ten minutes.

By necessity, we have become cautious sailors. We are less apt to go out if it is very windy or if the tide is low (as the ramp to our dock will be too steep). Chores that Tom would routinely perform around the house are also problematic. For example, he wanted to repair a damaged wire to the TV antennae. After much discussion, I climbed the ladder and attempted to strip the wires, while Tom instructed from below. In my new role as Tom's sidekick on sea and land, I vacillate between feeling terrified and exhilarated. I am also in awe of his determination to do as much as possible. When he rides the lawn mower sidesaddle, lugs wood from the shed, or ties a knot with one hand, I am reminded that he is resilient and resourceful.

When we recited our marriage vows thirty-two years ago, Tom and I had little understanding of unconditional love. This experience has deepened our love for one another, for our children and for our extended family and friends. It has made me more patient. I am a better listener. While there is a river of sadness running through our lives—a sense that the future we had planned might never be—there is also a growing confidence that we will not just survive this crisis, but move beyond it. I like to think that a year from now, Tom's stroke will no longer define and overshadow us; rather, it will have been the catalyst that pushed us to find new direction and meaning in our lives.

Gretchen TenBrook and Her Grandmother

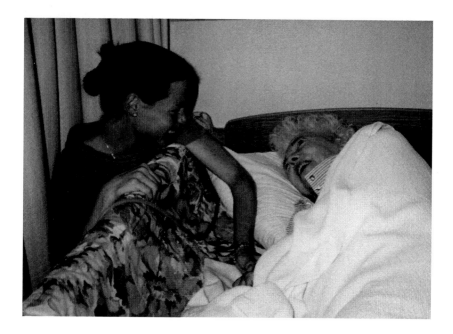

Author's photo

Good-Bye, Grandmère

By Gretchen TenBrook

Gretchen TenBrook has been an adjunct chaplain in the Department of Pastoral Care at the Johns Hopkins Hospital in Baltimore, Maryland. Her book, Broken Bodies, Healing Hearts, *vividly describes Gretchen's memories of her grandmother who had Alzheimer's.*

Alzheimer's is a devastating disease that causes progressive, incurable loss of memory. The incidence of Alzheimer's has increased dramatically now that our life expectancy has been prolonged. It begins with brief episodes of confusion, inability to drive in traffic, or a forgotten name and then progresses to complete helplessness. Friends and family can no longer be recognized. Caring for a loved one with Alzheimer's is emotionally stressful for the family and very expensive. New approaches in the care of people with Alzheimer's help them stay active and feel productive. These activities keep them busy with gardens, music and support groups that improve self-respect and dignity.

The thought of a baby had never come to mind when thinking about my grandmother. But that's exactly what popped into my head when I stood at her bedside on that late summer day at the nursing home. She lay curled up in a fetal position with the covers tucked firmly around her. Her freshly washed face appeared moist and rosy, yet expressionless, and her mouth quivered with occasional whimpers. I felt threatened by the fragile state of her withering condition.

The Grandmère who lay in front of me that day was not the Grandmère of my memories, however. I longed for the real Grandmère— the one who took me to Arch Cape for weekends at the beach; the one who ironed my grandfather's shirts while watching *One Life to Live* and sipping her afternoon cup of Kava; the one who fed the crusts of her morning toast to Smuckers, the faithful black Lab; the one who baked what seemed a thousand tins of Norwegian lefse for family and friends at Christmastime. But the Grandmère I knew was gone, ransacked by a thief called Alzheimer's disease. The dreaded diagnosis had progressed quickly, leaving her mind a prisoner to her body, a body that until recently had functioned as if it were twenty years younger. But now, the disease process was infesting her entire being. Her speech consisted of mere gibberish. Her arms and legs shook in brief and regular pulses. She wore diapers, too.

I don't visit my grandmother very often, about once every couple of years; she and I live on opposite coasts. Each time I see her, I am amazed by how her condition has deteriorated. It started back when I was in high school when one day she phoned in tears. Lost downtown with an armful of shopping bags, she was unable to remember where she had parked the old silver Volvo. I remember how terrified she was, not about losing her car, but about what the incident suggested about her. She mentioned nothing of this, but her unbridled tears and fidgeting fingers said it all; she dreaded what was to come and feared the inevitable conclusion.

The phone calls became more frequent, yet their pleas for help progressed from mere statements of fear to those of anger. "Why did you leave without telling me?" she would shriek in the midst of a hallucination. "But, Grandmère, we were never there," I would begin, only to hear the line click at the other end. Grandmère was not interested in answers that didn't make sense to her, in answers that only served to confirm the dementia she so deeply feared. To scream and yell in outrage, to blame everyone and anything around her, this was the only control she had on her world, a world she could no longer trust.

After Grandmère regularly began leaving the stove on and climbing into bed at ten o'clock in the morning, my family decided it was time to move her to an assisted-living center. Grandmère experienced it as another assault on her independence, further proof that she really was "going crazy."

The moving day is vivid in my memory. With my parents gently leading her arm-in-arm into the facility, she was initially quite content and, in fact, intrigued with the lovely building and its pristine surrounding landscape. However, when she saw her name written on an apartment door and realized she was to live there, her serenity turned to protest. She broke her arms loose and threw her purse violently across the room. Several other residents sitting in the living room stared listlessly at her. Soon Grandmère would react to her new neighbors the same way.

Now, as I stood at Grandmère's bedside years later, all of those memories flooded my mind like a tidal wave, a sharp contrast to the stillness of her present state. Lying motionless on the bed, seemingly void of any thought or emotion, she reminded me of a frozen computer screen indefinitely stuck in a state of nothingness. Would it not be better if she just shut down? This question left me with a sense of guilt that gnawed at me like a bleeding ulcer. "Do I really want my own grandmother to die?" I remember thinking to myself. In many ways, it seemed she already had.

In an attempt to make a connection—any connection—with Grandmère, I caressed her hand hoping it would awaken her from her slumber. Her eyes slowly cracked open and she turned her face from the pillow, looking right through me and gently giggling. 1 wanted to make eye contact with her. It seemed this was the only means of genuine relationship left; exchanging words of love and care or embracing in an intimate hug were no longer options.

"Hi, Grandmère," I uttered in a soft yet cheerful voice, kneeling at her bedside and smiling into her vacant eyes. "Remember me? I'm Gretchen, Terry's daughter." I knew my words made little sense to her, but I hoped that the tender way in which I tried to offer them would provide a loving message that even she could understand.

Apparently, she did understand the message. To my delight, she gazed directly into my eyes and whispered, "Oh, yes." Beaming with unspeakable joy, she appeared to be savoring the rare moment of togetherness that her disjointed world almost never allowed. Yes, the real Grandmère was back, even if only briefly. The precious moment came and went quickly, lasting no more than ten seconds. I sense that I will never truly see Grandmère again in this world. In that respect, the momentary bond with which we were blessed was as much of a greeting as it was a farewell, as much of a hello as it was a good-bye. The next time I see her, if there is a next time, the Alzheimer's will likely take another bite out of her being, leaving the landscape of her life even more barren than it already is. Receding further into infancy, she will become more and more like a baby. But instead of growing in her interaction with and attachment to the world, she will be finally set free from it.

Robert Horn

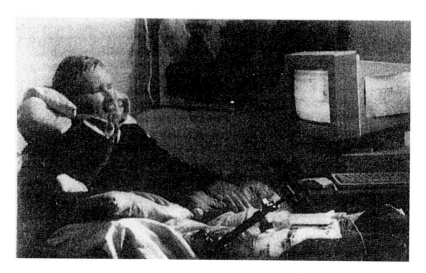

Photo by Ricardo De Aratanha

"It is frustrating...to be so absolutely helpless, but I am convinced that what I have left is more valuable than what I have lost... All in all, I would say that the glass has lost some of its water, but it is still half full." — Robert Horn

How Will They Know If I'm Dead?

By Robert Horn

Robert Horn is a father, soccer coach and gifted history teacher who has Amyo-
trophic Lateral Sclerosis (ALS), also known as Lou Gehrig's disease. This crippling
neuromuscular disease causes severe, progressive muscle weakness that is usually fatal in
three to five years. Horn recounts how he was diagnosed with ALS and his very personal
view on choosing life support in a book entitled How Will They Know If I'm Dead?
While he describes what it is like to be so utterly helpless, he also describes his optimism
and reveals his sense of humor. Horn's triumphant and inspiring book is dedicated to his
wife Judy.

I coached youth soccer for 15 years and I absolutely loved it. Impressed with the concept of the game of soccer as a metaphor for life, I
developed a little homily that became an integral part of my pre-game ora-
tory. "Soccer is like life. It doesn't matter how often you get knocked down
or if you lose the ball or make a mistake. Those things happen to each of
us. What does matter is whether and how quickly you recover, learn from
the experience and get back in the game. That's the test of character."

Somehow, when you are delivering such inspirational pronounce-
ments, you are not thinking of yourself but, rather, in terms of your audi-
ence. At least that was true in my case…So it was that I was unprepared to
apply my little bit of homespun philosophy to my own life in a big-time
way. All that changed on one sunny Friday afternoon in June 1988: I was
given a death sentence.

On that horrific day, I was told that I had Lou Gehrig's disease,
known medically as Amyotrophic Lateral Sclerosis or ALS. The diagnosis
came out of the blue. I went into the neurologist's office with a minor
twitch in my left arm and came out with a fatal motor neuron disease. My
world was suddenly turned upside-down. ALS is a particularly nasty disease
that kills you gradually, progressively, by blocking the messages from the
brain to the muscles. Within just a few years, often less than two, the muscles atrophy to the point of total paralysis. This paralysis includes the muscles that control swallowing and, most essential to life, breathing…ALS
leaves the mind intact so it can observe this steady physical deterioration.

I have been coping, battling if you prefer, with ALS for just over seven years. I have had virtually no functioning muscles for five years. I can't eat, speak or move. And I have been hooked to a ventilator for the past four-and-a-half years. That machine breathes for me. Everything I do takes a great deal of time. Communicating is especially slow. I "speak" with my eyebrows and spelling out every word, letter by letter is a tedious and lengthy process. About five hours of each of my days are consumed by necessary medical attention, getting bathed and dressed, taking a nap and, finally, being transported out to the living room where my computer waits with considerably more patience than its eager user. On my good days, I am usually able to work for five or six hours before I get too tired. I type with the only part of my body that I can move, my right foot, and this is another slow process. It takes me, on average, almost two days to type a page. Everything is a project.

It is frustrating and maddening to be so absolutely helpless and so totally dependent on others. If my head lolls to one side or the other, as it often does, it stays there unless and until someone notices and props it up again. If an arm slips off the armrest of the wheelchair, it will just dangle by my side until someone retrieves it.

There is more to life than physical ability. There are mental, emotional, and spiritual abilities or worlds to consider as well. In these worlds, I haven't changed: I am still a vibrant, healthy, and independent person. I can think, reason and analyze, remember, read, write, learn and communicate. I can love, feel happiness and sadness, be enthusiastic, get angry, have highs and lows, feel joy. I can believe, hope and have faith. That adds up to an extensive list of things that I can still "do" in spite of my disease.

This brings me back to the question of my overall perspective of my situation. I am convinced that what I have left is more valuable than what I have lost. I believe that the things I can do are more important than those I can't. The key for my psychological well-being is to focus on what I can do, my abilities, rather than on my disabilities and limitations. To dwell on the latter is to wallow in grief and self-pity. Such wallowing is, for me, sometimes unavoidable and occasionally even necessary. But to concentrate on the former is to invite optimism, achievement, and new opportunities. All in all, I would say that the glass has lost some of its water but it is still half full.

Choosing to remain on a ventilator for life support is a very personal life-or-death decision for Robert Horn. He turned down a painless assisted-suicide opportunity because he feels life is worth living. However, he acknowledges that this might not be the right decision for everyone in his situation. By choosing to go on the ventilator, he renewed his faith in life.

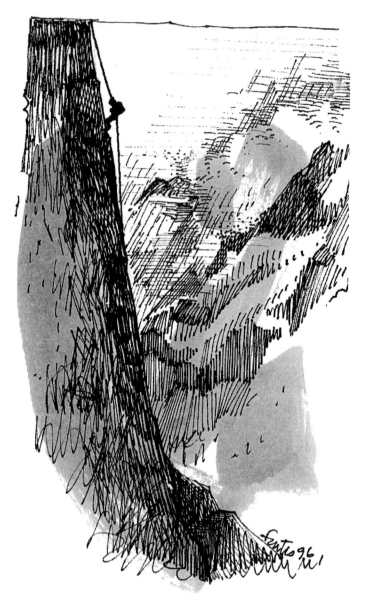

Illustrated by Larry Frates

Never Give Up!

Section III. Living Fully

Courage

The Endless Climb

By Dag Hammarskjold

The author served as secretary-general of the United Nations and was awarded the 1961 Nobel Peace Prize after his death in a plane crash. He wrote a book of poetry, prose and prayer entitled Markings *and loved climbing mountains. We need courage to overcome hardships. Courage is the ability to overcome hardships. Courage is the ability to keep going forward in spite of pain and suffering as described in this quotation and adjacent "Never Give Up!" illustration.*

When the morning's freshness

has been replaced by the weariness of midday,

when the leg muscles quiver under the strain,

the climb seems endless, and suddenly

nothing will go quite as you wish—it is

then that you must *not* hesitate.

Finding Hope & Compassion

George Gray, The Unfurled Sail

By Edgar Lee Masters, from *Spoon River Anthology*

This fictitious epitaph for a tombstone is explained by the dead George Gray himself, who describes his life and the meaning of the unfurled sail:

I have studied many times

The marble which was chiseled for me—

A boat with a furled sail at rest in a harbor.

In truth it pictures not my destination, but my life.

For love was offered me,

And I shrank from its disillusionment.

Sorrow knocked at my door, but I was afraid.

Ambition called for me, but I dreaded the chance,

Yet all the while I hungered for more meaning in my life.

And now I know that we must lift the sail

And catch the winds of destiny

Wherever they drive the boat.

To put meaning in one's life may end in madness,

But life without meaning is the torture

Of restlessness and vague desire—

It is a boat longing for the sea and yet afraid.

> Learn as if you were to live forever,
> Live as if you would die tomorrow.

– Isadore, Archbishop of Seville

The Man in the Arena

By Theodore Roosevelt

Theodore Roosevelt led a strenuous life and possessed great energy and courage, becoming President of the United States at age 42. His activities included hiking, hunting, horseback riding, swimming, and tennis. This remarkable man was also an author, conservationist, and statesman. Roosevelt received the Nobel Prize for peace in 1906, becoming the first American to win a Nobel Prize.

It is not the critic who counts, not the man who points out how the strong man stumbles or where the doer of deeds could have done them better. The credit belongs to the man who is actually in the arena, whose face is marred by dust and sweat and blood, who strives valiantly, who errs and comes short again and again because there is no effort without error and shortcomings, who knows the great devotion, who spends himself in a worthy cause, who at best knows in the end the high achievement of triumph and who at worst, if he fails while daring greatly, knows his place shall never be with those timid and cold souls who know neither victory nor defeat.

The Station

By Robert J. Hastings

This message by Reverend Hastings is full of youthful exuberance and urges us to seize the moment. Overcome fear, accept responsibility, reach out to help others! Do it now before it is too late! Love, laugh, sing for joy! "Life must be lived as we go along." Our reward will come soon enough.

Tucked away in our subconscious minds is an idyllic vision in which we see ourselves on a long journey that spans an entire continent. We're traveling by train and, from the windows, we drink in the passing scenes of cars on nearby highways, of children waving at crossings, of cattle grazing in distant pastures, of smoke pouring from power plants, of row upon row of corn and cotton and wheat, of flatlands and valleys, of city skylines and village halls.

But uppermost in our minds is our final destination–for at a certain hour and on a given day, our train will finally pull into the station with bells ringing, flags waving, and bands playing. And once that day comes, so many wonderful dreams will come true. So restlessly, we pace the aisles and count the miles, peering ahead, waiting, waiting, waiting for the station.

"Yes, when we reach the station, that will be it!" we promise ourselves.

"When we're eighteen...win that promotion...put the last kid through college...buy that 450 SL Mercedes Benz...pay off the mortgage...have a nest egg for retirement."

From that day on we will all live happily ever after.

Sooner or later, however, we must realize there is no station in this life, no one earthly place to arrive at once and for all. The journey is the joy...The station is an illusion–it constantly outdistances us. Yesterday's a memory, tomorrow's a dream. Yesterday belongs to a history, tomorrow belongs to God. Yesterday's a fading sunset, tomorrow's a faint moonrise. Only today is there light enough to love and live.

So, gently close the door on yesterday and throw the key away. It isn't the burdens of today that drive men mad, but rather the regret over yesterday and the fear of tomorrow.

"Relish the moment" is a good motto, especially when coupled with Psalm 118:24, "This is the day which the Lord hath made; we will rejoice and be glad in it."

So stop pacing the aisles and counting the miles. Instead, swim more rivers, climb more mountains, kiss more babies, count more stars. Laugh more and cry less. Go barefoot oftener. Eat more ice cream. Ride more merry-go-rounds. Watch more sunsets. Life must be lived as we go along.

Finding Hope & Compassion

Courage, Gaiety, and the Quiet Mind

By Robert Louis Stevenson

This master storyteller died at age 44 of tuberculosis on the South Sea island of Samoa. He shared his faith by composing prayers for the Samoan people. His kindness won the affection of the natives who built a road to his house called "The Road of the Loving Heart."

Give us courage, gaiety, and the quiet
mind. Spare to us our friends, soften
to us our enemies. Bless us, if it may be,
in all our innocent endeavors. If it may
not, give us the strength to encounter
that which is to come, that we be
brave in peril, constant in tribulation,
temperate in wrath, and in all changes
of fortune and down to the gates of
death, loyal, and loving to one another.

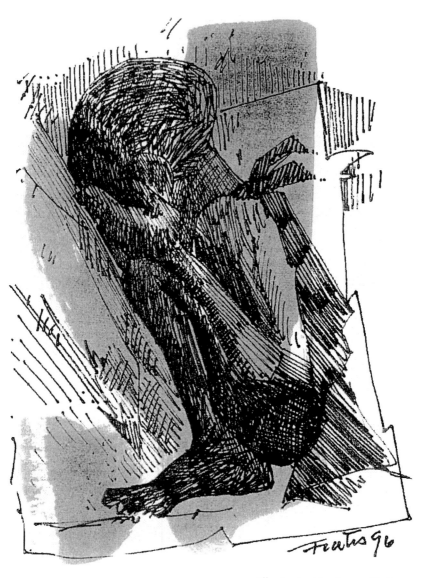

Illustrated by Larry Frates

Why Have You Forsaken Me?

Suffering & Caring

A Creed for Those Who Have Suffered

By an Unknown Confederate Soldier

Roy Campanella was a great Brooklyn Dodger baseball catcher who became a quadriplegic with paralysis of all four extremities following a spinal cord injury. In an article for the book Chicken Soup for the Soul by Canfield and Hansen, Campanella describes reading a bronze plaque at the Institute of Physical Medicine and Rehabilitation in New York that inspired him with the faith to accept his disability. The eloquent words on this plaque have been attributed to an unknown Confederate soldier.

I asked God for strength, that I might achieve.

    I was made weak, that I might learn humbly to obey…

I asked for health, that I might do greater things.

    I was given infirmity, that I might do better things…

I asked for riches, that I might be happy.

    I was given poverty, that I might be wise…

I asked for power, that I might have the praise of men.

    I was given weakness, that I might feel the need of God…

I asked for all things, that I might enjoy life.

    I was given life, that I might enjoy all things…

I got nothing I asked for—but everything I had hoped for.

    Almost despite myself, my unspoken prayers were answered.

    I am, among men, most richly blessed!

Living Fully Until Death

By Morrie Schwartz

What is it like to have a loved one facing death? Morrie Schwartz was a Professor of Sociology at Brandeis University. He developed ALS, or Lou Gehrig's disease, a disorder characterized by progressive muscle weakness that ultimately causes death. Morrie struggled to find meaning as he faced the unknown. Is it possible to accept death and still enjoy life? Sharing his thoughts about suffering with loved ones was comforting and helped him say goodbye. Surrounded by family and friends, he knew that he was loved and not alone. These thoughts were recorded in a taped audiovisual interview by the Department of Visual Media at the Dartmouth-Hitchcock Medical Center for the "Doctor Is In" series. (Reference: Tuesdays with Morrie *by Mitch Albom.)*

Talk openly about illness.
If you hide it, it is only going to be worse…
If you close yourself off…
Or make yourself tight because you
want to hold in all these horrible feelings,
it will only get worse.
Open yourself up as much as you can.

There's this constant dynamic tension between opposites—

I'm a child, I'm an adult.
I want to live, I want to die.
I love and I'm not so loving.
Where is the balance?

There is more to this life than just
a concrete hard phenomenon.
Is that all there is, birth and death,
a mechanical process?
There are a lot of mysteries
that one ponders about,
especially the one about death,
which I can't answer.

Renewal of Spiritual Strength

By Rabbi Harold S. Kushner

When Rabbi Kushner's son died at age 14 of a rare disease, Kushner wondered why innocent people had to suffer. After the death of a loved one, a safe harbor is needed to rest, heal wounds, forgive mistakes, share memories, and celebrate the courage and compassion of those we love. The poet Sophocles wrote, "One must wait until evening to see how splendid the day has been." Each person is unique. When we look back upon the life of a loved one, we can say that life has indeed been splendid.

This compassionate insight is a source of comfort in times of grief and helps us realize that we are not alone in our suffering.

Where do you get the strength to go on, when you have used up all of your own strength?

Where do you turn for patience when you have run out of patience, when you have been more patient than anyone should be asked to be, and the end is nowhere in sight?

I believe that God gives us strength and patience and hope, renewing our spiritual resources when they run dry.

Finding Hope & Compassion

Bless Night Nurses

By Paul Wiggin

Paul Wiggin is the director of the inspirational singing group MUSE (Music Serving Elders).

This poem is also a song that records Paul's journey from despair to hope, following his first major surgery. The quotation that follows explains his feelings, "I was afraid I'd die on the operating table, or that they would find it was too late for successful surgery, which happened forty years ago to my uncle. But, hey, a miracle happened and this time it was successful!

I returned home after eight days in the hospital, renewed inside and out, healed in more ways than one by the skill and dedication of gifted miracle workers who restored my life and hope. How can I keep from singing praises to all, especially my kind, unflappable nurses who relieved my pain and loneliness during the long, dark nights in the hospital?"

how many came to heal me
the Lord could better say
whose angels saw me falling
in the vale of yesterday

i don't know where they came from
i only know they came
around the clock till dawn was up
in the vale of yesterday

thankful for the morning light
purged of all the pain
each face and conversation bright
i treasure and retain

their art and dedication
has led me to this day
past the dark and trepidation
of the vale of yesterday

All in a Day's Work

By Naomi Rhode

A compassionate nurse renews hope in a sick man who feels lonely and neglected.

Emergency-room personnel transported him to the cardiac floor. Long hair, unshaven, dirty, dangerously obese and a black motorcycle jacket tossed on the bottom shelf of the stretcher—an outsider to this sterile world of shining terrazzo floors, efficient uniformed professionals and strict infection-control procedures.

Definitely an untouchable!

The nurses at the station looked wide-eyed as this mound of humanity was wheeled by—each glancing nervously at my friend Bonnie, the head nurse. "Let this one not be mine to admit, bathe and tend to..." was the pleading, unspoken message from their inner concern.

One of the true marks of a leader, a consummate professional, is to do the unthinkable. To touch the untouchable. To tackle the impossible. Yes, it was Bonnie who said, "I want this patient myself." Highly unusual for a head nurse—unconventional—but "the stuff" out of which human spirits thrive, heal and soar. As she donned her latex gloves and proceeded to bathe this huge, filthy man, her heart almost broke. Where was his family? Who was his mother? What was he like as a little boy?

She hummed quietly as she worked to ease the fear and embarrassment she knew he must have been feeling. And then on a whim she said, "We don't have time for back rubs much in hospitals these days, but I bet one would really feel good. And, it would help you relax your muscles and start to heal. That is what this place is all about—a place to heal."

All in a day's work. Touching the untouchable.

His thick, scaly, ruddy skin told a story of an abusive lifestyle. Probably lots of addictive behavior, to food, alcohol and drugs. As Bonnie rubbed the taut muscles, she hummed and prayed. Prayed for the soul of a little boy grown up, rejected by life's rudeness and striving for acceptance in a hard, hostile world.

The finale—warmed lotion and baby powder. Almost laughable—such a contrast on this huge, rugged surface. As he rolled over onto his back, tears rolled down his cheek. With amazingly beautiful brown eyes, he smiled and said in a quivering voice, "No one has touched me for years." His chin trembled. "Thank you. I *am* healing."

In a day when we have increasing concern about the appropriateness of touch, Bonnie taught this hurting world to still dare to touch the untouchable through eye contact, a warm handshake, a concerned voice—or the physical reassurance of warmed lotion and baby powder.

Death in the First Person

Anonymous

A dying student nurse shares her feelings about suffering and loneliness with other nurses, hoping that they will become more compassionate and able to care for the needs of the sick. Simple acts of kindness and listening are comforting. They show that we care.

I am a student nurse. I am dying. I write this to you who are, and will become nurses in the hope that by my sharing my feelings with you, you may someday be better able to help those who share my experience.

I'm out of the hospital now—perhaps for a month, for six months, perhaps for a year—but no one likes to talk about such things. In fact, no one likes to talk about much at all. Nursing must be advancing, but I wish it would hurry. We're taught not to be overly cheery now, to omit the "Everything's fine" routine, and we have done pretty well. But now one is left in a lonely silent void. With the protective "fine, fine" gone, the staff is left with only their own vulnerability and fear. The dying patient is not yet seen as a person and thus cannot be communicated with as such. He is a symbol of what every human fears and what we each know, at least academically, that we too must someday face. What did they say in psychiatric nursing about meeting pathology with pathology to the detriment of both patient and nurse? And there was a lot about knowing one's own feelings before you could help another with his. How true.

But for me, fear is today and dying is now. You slip in and out of my room, give me medications and check my blood pressure. Is it because I am a student nurse, myself, or just a human being, that I sense your fright? And your fears enhance mine. Why are you afraid? I am the one who is dying!

I know, you feel insecure, don't know what to say, don't know what to do. But please believe me, if you care, you can't go wrong. Just admit that you care. That is really for what we search. We may ask for why's and wherefore's, but we don't really expect answers. Don't run away—wait—all I want to know is that there will be someone to hold my hand when I need it. I am afraid. Death may get to be a routine to you, but it is new to me. You may not see me as unique, but I've never died before. To me, once is pretty unique!

You whisper about my youth, but when one is dying, is he really so young anymore? I have lots I wish we could talk about. It really would not take much more of your time because you are in here quite a bit anyway.

If only we could be honest, both admit of our fears, touch one another. If you really care, would you lose so much of your valuable professionalism if you even cried with me? Just person to person? Then, it might not be so hard to die—in a hospital—with friends close by.

Mother to Son

By Langston Hughes

*In this poem written by a gifted African American, a proud and courageous
mother urges her son not to give up when he faces adversity. Hughes wrote many plays
and poems and became a leader of the Harlem Renaissance during the 1920s.*

Well, son, I'll tell you:

Life for me ain't been no crystal stair.

It's had tacks in it,

And splinters,

And boards torn up,

And places with no carpet on the floor—

Bare.

But all the time,

I'se been a-climbin' on,

And reachin' landin's,

And turnin' corners,

And sometimes goin' in the dark

Where there ain't been no light.

So boy, don't you turn back.

Don't you set down on the steps

Cause you finds it's kinder hard.

Don't you fall now—

For I'se still goin', honey,

I'se still climbin',

And life for me ain't been no crystal stair.

What God Has Promised

By Annie Johnson Flint

This eloquent poem helps us become more aware of our spiritual needs. Life is a precious gift and contains both joy and sorrow.

God has not promised skies always blue,

Flower-strewn pathways, all our lives through.

God has not promised

    Sun without rain,

    Joy without sorrow,

    Peace without pain:

But God has promised

    Strength for the day,

    Rest for our labor,

    Light for the way,

    Grace for our trials,

    Help from above,

    Unfailing sympathy,

    Undying love.

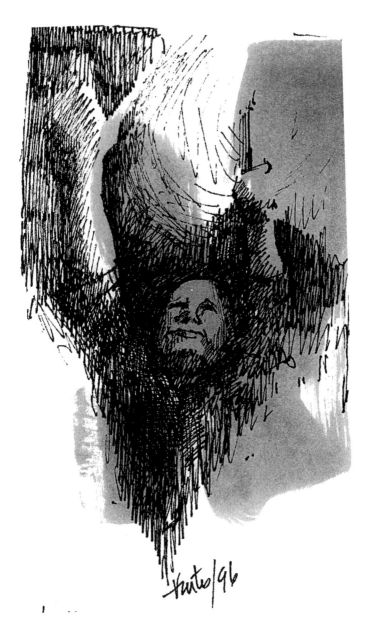

Illustrated by Larry Frates

It's better to light one small candle than to curse the darkness.
(A favorite quotation of Eleanor Roosevelt and Adlei Stevenson)

Hope & Faith

Without This Faith

By Helen Keller

Deaf and blind since age one and one-half, Helen Keller learned to speak, read, and write through the sense of touch. Her faith guided her through the darkness, helping her to become an inspiring speaker and author.

Without this faith
there would be little meaning in my life,
I should be
"a mere pillar of darkness in the dark."

Observers in the full enjoyment
of their bodily senses pity me,
but it is because
they do not see
the golden chamber in my life
where I dwell delighted;
for, dark as my path may seem to them,
I carry a magic light in my heart.

Faith,
the spiritual strong searchlight,
illumines the way,
and although sinister doubts lurk in the shadow,
I walk unafraid
towards the Enchanted Wood
where the foliage is always green,
where joy abides,
where nightingales nest and sing,
and where life and death are one
in the presence of the Lord.

The Road Ahead

By Thomas Merton

This beloved spiritual writer became a Catholic Trappist priest. He led a strict monastic religious life. Merton's writings on the inward journey of solitude help us to share his struggle for greater love and humility, revealing his warmth and inner joy. His autobiography, The Seven Story Mountain, *won wide acclaim.*

My Lord, God, I have no idea where I am going. I do not see the road ahead of me. I cannot know for certain where it will end. Nor do I really know myself, and the fact that I think I am following your will does not mean that I am actually doing so. But I believe that the desire to please You does in fact please You. And I hope I have that desire in all that I am doing. I hope that I will never do anything apart from the desire. And I know that if I do this, you will lead me by the right road, though I may know nothing about it. Therefore will I trust You always though I may seem to be lost in the shadow of death. I will not fear for You are ever with me, and you will never leave me to face my perils alone.

Irish Blessing

Author Unknown

May the road rise to meet you,

May the wind be always at your back.

May the sun shine warm upon your face,

The rains fall softly upon your fields,

And, until we meet again,

May God hold you in the palm of his hand.

Serenity Prayer

By Reinhold Niebuhr

This influential theologian taught religion at the Union Theological Seminary in New York City and is known for his books on Christian ethics. His serenity prayer is used by members of Alcoholics Anonymous to begin AA meetings and inspire discussion groups.

God grant me the serenity
to accept the things
I cannot change,
courage to change the things
I can, and the wisdom
to know the difference.

Living one day at a time;
Enjoying one moment at a time;
Accepting hardship as the
pathway to peace.

Taking, as He did, this sinful world
As it is, not as I would have it;
Trusting that He will make all things
right if I surrender to His will;

That I may be reasonably happy
in this life,
And supremely happy with Him
forever in the next.

Make Me an Instrument of Thy Peace

By Saint Francis of Assisi

Giovanni Bernardine, known today as Saint Francis, was born in Assisi, Italy. He founded the Franciscans, a Roman Catholic religious order devoted to the care of the sick and poor. Fondly remembered for his love of nature and all living things, he has been named the patron saint of ecology.

At age twenty, Francis was taken prisoner for a year in a battle against a neighboring city. Afterwards he suffered from illness, had an encounter with a leper, and underwent a religious conversion that transformed him from a wealthy young man into a poor missionary. He renounced all his belongings, dedicated his life to God, and lived in poverty. Often sick and near starvation, Francis died in 1226 at the age of forty-five. He was declared a saint, canonized, two years after his death.

Lord, make me an instrument of Thy peace;
where there is hatred, let me sow love;
where there is injury, pardon;
where there is doubt, faith;
where there is despair, hope;
where there is darkness, light;
and where there is sadness, joy.

O Divine Master, grant that I may not so much seek
to be consoled, as to console;
to be understood, as to understand;
to be loved, as to love;
for it is in giving that we receive,
in pardoning that we are pardoned,
and in dying, we are born to eternal life.

All Things Bright and Beautiful

By Cecil Frances Alexander

Mrs. Alexander wrote many religious hymns for children in the nineteenth century. Her husband became Primate of all Ireland. The delightful words of this hymn were used by the British veterinarian, James Herriot, in the titles of four books describing his practice in Yorkshire, England.

All things bright and beautiful,
    All creatures great and small,
All things wise and wonderful,
    The Lord God made them all.
Each little flower that opens,
    Each little bird that sings,
He made their glowing colours,
    He made their tiny wings.
The purple-headed mountain,
    The river running by,
The sunset, and the morning
    That brightens up the sky.
The cold wind in the winter,
    The pleasant summer sun,
The ripe fruits in the garden,
    He made them everyone.
The tall trees in the greenwood,
    The meadows where we play,
The rushes by the water
    We gather every day.
He gave us eyes to see them,
    And lips that we might tell
How great is God Almighty
    Who has made all things well.

Look to This Day

By Kalidasa

Translated from Sanskrit, Fifth Century A.D., India

Listen to the exhortation of the dawn!
Look to this day!
For it is life, the very life of life.
In its brief course lie all the verities
And realities of your existence:

> The bliss of growth,
>
> The glory of action,
>
> The splendor of beauty;

For yesterday is but a dream,
And tomorrow is only a vision;
But today, well-lived, makes every yesterday

> A dream of happiness,

And every tomorrow a vision of hope.
Look well, therefore, to this day.
Such is the salutation of the dawn.

Epilogue

The Good, the Bad, and the Wonderful

The true stories in this book may help us look into our own blind spots and see ourselves and others in a new light. What really counts in life is how we treat one another. Generosity, a sense of humor, and compassion improve relationships and bring people closer together. It is always difficult to be concerned about other people's problems when we are already worried about our own. If we see a woman in a wheelchair who needs help, would we stop and offer assistance or pretend that we don't see her? Arthur Gordon, in his book *A Touch of Wonder*, enjoys telling how his Boy Scout troop leader would warn them, "Don't be a buttoned-up person. Stop wearing your raincoat in the shower." He hoped they would always be kind, live life with enthusiasm, and not be afraid of new experiences.

Facing reality is not always a pleasant task. We all have moments of doubt when we need to cling to something worthwhile. Too often we shuffle into the future without enough hope, perhaps alone, and overburdened. It is the gift of the poet to help us see there is a certain dignity and grandeur in life itself. We need to be reminded of lasting values such as love, hope, and courage that can renew our strength, helping us to push forward in the midst of uncertainty.

We also need respect and the knowledge that what we do matters, that our life has meaning. Ralph Waldo Emerson wrote the following list of qualities that can make life worthwhile.

Success

To laugh often and much;

To win the respect of intelligent people
    and the affection of children;

To earn the appreciation of honest critics
    and endure the betrayal of false friends;

To appreciate beauty; to find the best in others;

To leave the world a bit better,
>   whether by a healthy child,
>   a garden patch
>   or a redeemed social condition;

To know even one life has breathed easier
>   because you have lived.

This is to have succeeded.

Anyone who has given and received love and kindness knows that life can have unexpected moments of joy and meaning. People who are in trouble become grateful for anything that we can do for them. Kindness is never wasted. We are at our best when struggling against pain, ignorance, and fear.

How can we give comfort and renew hope in people who are sick or discouraged, and have no more strength left to keep on going? The words in the songs that follow may give them a second wind, a wind beneath their wings helping them to soar upwards with confidence, helping them to know that they are still loved and not all alone. Please don't hesitate to sing along while reading these lyrics.

Ludwig van Beethoven's Ninth Symphony glorifies the brotherhood of mankind and ends with a feeling of great joy and optimism. Beethoven was totally deaf when he wrote the Ninth Symphony. The final movement includes an inspiring ode to joy written by Friedrich Schiller, a famous German writer and poet. Beethoven's Ninth Symphony is often listed now in hymnbooks as "Joyful, Joyful, We Adore Thee." The first two verses of the final movement are written below.

Joyful, Joyful, We Adore Thee

Joyful, joyful, we adore thee, God of Glory, Lord of love;
Hearts unfold like flowers before thee, opening to the sun above.
Melt the clouds of sin and sadness, drive the dark of doubt away.
Giver of immortal gladness, fill us with the light of day!
All thy works with joy surround thee, earth and heav'n reflect thy rays,
Stars and angels sing around thee, center of unbroken praise.
Field and forest, vale and mountain, flowery meadow, flashing sea,
Chanting bird and flowing fountain, call us to rejoice in thee.

The moving spiritual song that follows has been sung by slaves and other unfortunate people who hoped for a better life in heaven. It is a beautiful description of unconditional love. The lyrics were written by the Irish poet Thomas Moore, who lived from 1779-1852. Many of his words have been set to music.

"Come, ye disconsolate, where'er ye languish,
Come to the mercy seat, fervently kneel;
Here bring your wounded hearts, here tell your anguish;
Earth hath no sorrow that heaven cannot heal.

Joy of the desolate, Light of the straying,
Hope of the penitent, fadeless and pure!
Here speaks the Comforter, tenderly saying.
'Earth hath no sorrow that heaven cannot cure.'

Here see the Bread of Life; see waters flowing
Forth from the throne of God; pure from above;
Come to the feast of love; come, ever knowing
Earth hath no sorrow but heaven can remove."

The day breaks and the shadows flee away.

—Fra Giovanni MDXIII

Share Your Thoughts

The editors of this book are interested in hearing from you. We find that these stories move people in different ways. If you would like to share your thoughts about this book with the us, we would be very grateful.

Contact us through email in care of editor Carolyn Charron:

CCharron@partners.org

Permissions

Anonymous. "Death in the First Person." *American Journal of Nursing* Volume 70, Issue 2 (February 1970): 336-338.

Armstrong, Lance, with Sally Jenkins. *It's Not About the Bike: My Journey Back to Life*. New York: G. P. Putnam's Sons, 2000. Excerpt from "Chemo," from *It's Not About the Bike* by Lance Armstrong, copyright © 2000 by Lance Armstrong. Used by permission of G.P. Putnam's Sons, and division of Penguin Group (USA) Inc.

Berg, Art. "To the Top." *Guideposts* (April 2002). Reprinted with permission from *Guideposts* magazine. Copyright © 2002 by *Guideposts*. All rights reserved. www.guidepostsmag.com

Brinckerhoff, Constance. "The Winter of Our Discontent." *Dartmouth Medicine* (Winter 1998).

Buscaglia, Leo. *Born for Love: Reflections on Loving*. Thorofare, NJ: SLACK Incorporated, 1992. Reprinted with permission from SLACK Incorporated.

Coles, Robert. *The Moral Intelligence of Children*. New York: Plume, 1997. From *The Moral Intelligence of Children* by Robert Coles, copyright © 1997 Robert Coles. Used by permission of Random House, Inc.

Cousins, Norman. *Anatomy of an Illness as Perceived by the Patient*. New York: W. W. Norton & Company, 1979. From *Anatomy of an Illness as Perceived by the Patient: Reflections on Healing and Regeneration* by Norman Cousins. Copyright © 1979 by W. W. Norton & Company, Inc. Used by permission of W. W. Norton & Company, Inc.

Donnelly, John. "I'm One of Six Children. I'm the Only One Left." *The Boston Globe* (January 26, 2003).

Ehrmann, Max. "Desiderata." © 1927 by Max Ehrmann. Used by permission of Bell & Son Publishing, LLC. All rights reserved.

Flannery, Margaret. "Courage Is in the Eye of the Beholder." Permission for publication given by Margaret Flannery.

Foley, Anne. "Regaining What's Been Lost." *Dartmouth Medicine* (Winter 2001).

Gilbert, Peggy. "The Impact of a Stroke on a Marriage." Permission for publication given by Peggy and Tom Gilbert.

Goldman, Jami, and Andrea Cagan. *Up and Running: The Jami Goldman Story*. New York: Atria Books, 2001. Reprinted and edited with the permission of Atria Books, a Division of Simon & Schuster, Inc., from

Up and Running: The Jami Goldman Story by Jami Goldman. Copyright © 2001 by Jami Goldman. All rights reserved.

Hammarskjold, Dag. *Markings.* New York: Knopf: 1966. From *Markings* by Dag Hammarskjold, translated by W. H. Auden and Leif Sjoberg, translation copyright © 1964, copyright renewed 1992 by Alfred A. Knopf, a division of Random House, Inc., and Faber & Faber Ltd. Foreword copyright © 1964 by W. H. Auden, copyright renewed 1992 by Edward Mendelson. Used by permission of Alfred A. Knopf, a division of Random House, Inc.

Hastings, Robert J. *A Penny's Worth of Minced Ham: Another Look at the Great Depression.* Carbondale: Southern Illinois University Press, 1986. From *A Penny's Worth of Minced Ham: Another Look at the Great Depression* by Robert Hastings. Copyright © 1986 by Southern Illinois University Press. Reprinted by permission of the publisher.

Hine, Robert V. *Second Sight.* Berkeley: University of California Press, 1993.

Horn, Robert C., III. *How Will They Know If I'm Dead?* Boca Raton: GR/St. Lucie Press, 1997.

Hughes, Langston. "Mother to Son." In *The Collected Poems of Langston Hughes,* edited by Arnold Rampersad with David Roessel. New York: Knopf, 1994. "Mother to Son," from *The Collected Poems of Langston Hughes* by Langston Hughes, edited by Arnold Rampersad with David Roessel, Associate Editor, copyright © 1994 by The Estate of Langston Hughes. Used by permission of Alfred A. Knopf, a division of Random House, Inc.

Iezzoni, Lisa I. "What Should I Say? Communication around Disability." *Annals of Internal Medicine* 129 (1998): 661-665.

Jamison, Kay Redfield. *An Unquiet Mind: A Memoir of Moods and Madness.* New York: Knopf, 1995. From *An Unquiet Mind* by Kay Redfield Jamison, copyright © 1995 by Kay Redfield Jamison. Used by permission of Alfred A. Knopf, a division of Random House, Inc.

Jamison, Kay Redfield. *Night Falls Fast: Understanding Suicide.* New York: Knopf, 1999. From *Night Falls Fast* by Kay Redfield Jamison, copyright © 1999 by Kay Redfield Jamison. Used by permission of Alfred A. Knopf, a division of Random House, Inc.

Keller, Helen. *Midstream: My Later Life.* New York: Doubleday, 1929. From *Midstream* by Helen Keller, copyright © 1929 by Helen Keller and The Crowell Publishing Company. Used by permission of Doubleday, a division of Random House, Inc.

Khan, Muhammad Asim. "On Being a Patient: The Patient-Doctor." *Annals of Internal Medicine* 133 (2000): 233-235.

Kushner, Harold S. *When Bad Things Happen to Good People*. New York: Schocken Books, 1981. From *When Bad Things Happen to Good People* by Harold S. Kushner, copyright © 1981 by Harold S. Kushner. Preface copyright © by Harold S. Kushner. Used by permission of Schocken Books, a division of Random House, Inc.

Last, Eric C. "On Being a Patient: For Corrie." *Annals of Internal Medicine* 124 (1996): 271-272.

Lee, Joshua, "Bring The Words Forward." *Dartmouth Medicine* (Fall 2001).

Masters, Edgar Lee. *Spoon River Anthology*. New York: Penguin Books, 1992.

McDavid, Lee. "Only clad with skin." Introductory Commentary to "Regaining What's Been Lost." *Dartmouth Medicine* (Winter 2001).

Merton, Thomas. *Thoughts in Solitude*. New York: Farrar, Straus & Giroux, 1958. "The Road Ahead" from "The Love of Solitude" from *Thoughts in Solitude* by Thomas Merton. Copyright © 1958 by the Abbey of Our Lady of Gethsemani. Copyright renewed 1986 by the Trustees of the Thomas Merton Legacy Trust. Reprinted by permission of Farrar, Straus and Giroux, LLC.

Miller, Dan, with Jeane Zornes. *Living, Laughing and Loving Life*. Mukilteo, WA: Wine Press Publishing, 1997.

Nutt, Robert. "Silence Is Sound." *Dartmouth Medicine* (2002).

O'Neil, Joseph. "Your Son Is Dying." In *AIDS Doctors: Voices from the Epidemic, An Oral History*, edited by Ronald Bayer and Gerald M. Oppenheimer. Oxford: Oxford University Press, 2000. Copyright © 2000 by Oxford University Press. Reprinted by permission of Oxford University Press. All rights reserved.

Proal, Cheryl. "Pain Is Inevitable, Misery Is Optional." Permission for publication given by Cheryl Proal.

Remen, Rachel Naomi. *Kitchen Table Wisdom: Stories That Heal*. New York: Riverhead Books 1996. "Just Listen," from *Kitchen Table Wisdom* by Rachel Naomi Remen, M.D., copyright © 1996 by Rachel Naomi Remen, M.D. Used by permission of Riverhead Books, an imprint of Penguin Group (USA) Inc.

Remen, Rachel Naomi. *My Grandfather's Blessings*. New York: Riverhead Books, 2000. "When Somebody Knows," from *My Grandfather's Blessings* by Rachel Naomi Remen, M.D., copyright © 2000 by Rachel Naomi Remen, M.D. Used by permission of Riverhead Books, an imprint of Penguin Group (USA) Inc.

Rhode, Naomi. "All in a Day's Work." In *Chicken Soup for the Nurse's Soul*. Deerfield Beach, FL: Health Communications Inc., 2001.

Rooney, Timothy. "One March Morning." *Dartmouth Medicine* (Spring 2003).

Sack, Burton. Introductory Commentary to "Courage Is in the Eye of the Beholder." Permission for publication given by Burton Sack, M.D.

Schwartz, Morrie. "Living Fully Until Death." Permission for publication given by Mrs. Charlotte Schwartz.

Selwyn, Peter. *Surviving the Fall: The Personal Journey of an AIDS Doctor.* New Haven, CT: Yale University Press, 1998. From *Surviving the Fall* by Peter Selwyn, copyright © 1998 by Peter Selwyn. Used by permission of Yale University Press.

Stair, Nadine. "If I Had My Life to Live Over." In *Chicken Soup for the Soul.* Deerfield Beach, FL: Health Communications, Inc., 1993.

TenBrook, Gretchen, and Harold G. Koenig. *Broken Bodies, Healing Hearts: Reflections of a Hospital Chaplain.* Binghamton, NY: Haworth Press, 2000. "Good-Bye, Grandmère," from *Broken Bodies, Healing Hearts* by Gretchen TenBrook and Harold G. Koenig, copyright © 2000 by Hawthorn Press. Reprinted by permission of Hawthorn Press. All rights reserved.

Warner, Gale, with David Kreger. *Dancing at the Edge of Life: A Memoir.* New York: Hyperion Books, 1998. From the book *Dancing at the Edge of Life* by Gale Warner. Copyright © 1998 David Kreger, M.D. Reprinted by permission of Hyperion. All rights reserved.

Wiggin, Paul. "Bless Night Nurses." Permission for publication given by Paul Wiggin.

About the Editors

William P. Beetham, Jr, MD

Dr. Beetham practiced medicine for over 40 years on staff at the Lahey Clinic, New England Deaconess Hospital, and Harvard Medical School until he retired. He received his degree in medicine from the University of Rochester, New York and completed post graduate training in medicine and rheumatology at the Boston City Hospital and the Mayo Clinic. He co-authored the widely accepted textbook, *Physical Examination of the Joints*, published by W.B. Saunders. Dr. Beetham has served as president of the New England Rheumatism Association and was voted best clinical teacher by the medical residents at the New England Deaconess Hospital.

He practiced compassionate medicine: "As I grew older, I became more aware of the emotional needs of my patients. There is a warm feeling that arises from giving and receiving kindness and respect. Love grows as it is shared. I realized that life is a precious gift and contains both joy and sorrow. In spite of pain and suffering, the resilience of the human spirit is a source of inspiration. We are never more heroic than when we search for the courage to overcome fear and ignorance."

Ellen Burke Ceppetelli, RN, MS, CNL

Ellen Burke Ceppetelli has been a nurse educator for 34 of 40 years in nursing. Currently, she is the director of nursing education at Dartmouth-Hitchcock Medical Center. In addition, she is an instructor in family and community medicine at Dartmouth Medical School where she collaborates with Dr. O'Donnell in teaching an enrichment elective that provides nurse shadowing experiences for first year medical students. She received her BSN from the University of Massachusetts, Amherst and MS in community health nursing from Boston College. Ellen was a visiting scholar for 18 years at the Harvard School of Public Health and now serves as chair of the board of advisors of the Harvard-NIOSH Education and Research Center for Occupational Safety and Health.

American Nurses Credentialing Center (ANCC) certified for 20 years in community health nursing, Ellen believes "the privileged intimacy that nurses share with patients and their families during illness and health is a unique gift that carries immense responsibility."

Carolyn Charron, BSN, RN, OCN

Carolyn Charron is Dr. Beetham's daughter and has been an oncology nurse for 25 years. She received a BSN from Duke University. She has worked at the University of Connecticut Health Center, Thompson Cancer Survival Center in Knoxville, Tennessee and for the past five years has been at the Dana Farber Cancer Institute in Boston, Massachusetts. She also worked as a hospice nurse for six years in both Knoxville, Tennessee and Cambridge, Massachusetts. Ms. Charron feels that creativity is an integral part of the healing process: "Creativity rejuvenates me. Finding the creative spark in my patients helps me form a deeper connection with them."

Joseph O'Donnell, MD

Dr. O'Donnell is a medical oncologist. He is professor of medicine and psychiatry, senior advising dean and director of community programs and senior scholar of the C Everett Koop Institute at Dartmouth Medical School where he has served for over 30 years. He is a former chief of oncology at the Dartmouth-affiliated White River Junction Veterans Administration Medical Center. He has served as president of the Northeast Group on Educational Affairs of the Association of American Medical Colleges and the American Association for Cancer Education and recipient of that latter organization's Margaret Hay Edwards Achievement Medal for his contributions to cancer education. He is a co-editor, along with Dr Robert Coles, Randy Testa, Penny Armstrong, and M Brownell Anderson of the book, *A Life in Medicine: A Literary Anthology*, published by The New Press, 2002.

Dr. O'Donnell believes that doctors can learn a great deal from the humanities and especially, from literature: "The stories of these great authors teach us how to listen carefully to the stories of our patients about their own dreams, hopes, and fears. I believe the heart of medicine is service for others. I try to give our students as many opportunities as I can to feel compassion, hoping they will seek out such chances in their lives as doctors."

Finding Hope & Compassion